MILK-BASED SOAPS

MAKING NATURAL, SKIN-NOURISHING SOAP

CASEY MAKELA

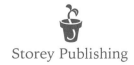

Storey Publishing

The mission of Storey Publishing is to serve our customers
by publishing practical information that encourages personal independence
in harmony with the environment.

Edited by Jenna Dixon
Cover design by Carol Jessop, Black Trout Design, and Susan Bernier
Cover art and interior spot illustrations by Laura Tedeschi; all other illustrations
    by Randy Mosher
Text design by Susan Bernier (based on an original design by Carol Jessop,
    Black Trout Design)
Text production by Jeff Potter, Potter Publishing Studio
Indexed by Susan Olason, Indexes & Knowledge Maps

© 1997 Storey Publishing, LLC

All rights reserved. No part of this book may be reproduced without written permission from the publisher, except by a reviewer who may quote brief passages or
reproduce illustrations in a review with appropriate credits; nor may any part of
this book be reproduced, stored in a retrieval system, or transmitted in any form
or by any means — electronic, mechanical, photocopying, recording, or other —
without written permission from the publisher.

The information in this book is true and complete to the best of our knowledge. All
recommendations are made without guarantee on the part of the author or Storey
Publishing. The author and publisher disclaim any liability in connection with the
use of this information. For additional information please contact Storey Publishing, 210 MASS MoCA Way, North Adams, MA 01247.

Storey books are available for special premium and promotional uses and for customized editions. For further information, please call 800-793-9396.

Printed in the United States by Edwards Brothers
10 9 8 7 6 5

Library of Congress Cataloging-in-Publication Data

Makela, Casey, 1960-
    Milk-based soaps : making natural, skin-nourishing soap / Casey Makela.
        p.   cm.
    Includes Index.
    ISBN 13: 978-0-88266-984-7; ISBN 10: 0-88266-984-2 (alk. paper)
    1. Soap.   2. Milk.   I. Title.
TP991.M27   1997
668'.124—dc21   97-30670
                                                                        CIP

TABLE OF CONTENTS

DEDICATION

*What joy in life could there ever be
without good friends and loving family?*

— Kimberly Ann Walker

My family patiently and lovingly allows me to be a writer and my good friends spur me on. I am forever grateful to them all.

To **William,** my beloved — thank you for your endless patience. You are so much more than just a husband. Your encouragement and support are a lifeline to me.

To my children: **Marion,** your beautiful freckle-faced smile illuminates my imagination. You are my rose in bloom. I love you. **John,** thank you for your bear hugs and sharing your dreams about tractors. I love my little "farmer man." **Patti,** thank you for making me laugh when I lose my sense of humor. I love you to the "Max." **Lori,** your motivation is an inspiration to me. I will always love my "Bubbles" and look forward to calling you Dr. Bubbles! **Sara,** my "Indian Woman." I love my darling girl. You are very special and a precious gem to me. **Dani,** you share my love of writing and I know you understand. I love you and we will travel through Europe together someday. **Wes,** you redefine humor and make us all laugh, and I love you for that. To all of you, thank you for being my children and giving me the joy of motherhood. You are my greatest accomplishments in life.

Mom — I know you are always there. Thank you for loving me when I need it most.

Maryanne — thank you for the many long hours you spent helping me, editing, and telling me I could. You are a gifted writer and a true friend.

Edie — your enthusiasm and joy for life are infectious. Thank you for making me feel special and being my friend.

Denise — thank you for showing me the lighter side of life and reminding me to laugh at impossible situations. Just keep the angel food cake coming!

Dean — thank you for baby-sitting me through the trials and errors of my first computer. I wish you great success with "I-STAR."

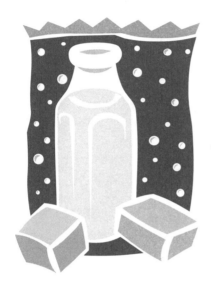

A Glance Back

CHAPTER 1

There is nothing in this world
except the history you do not know.
—Harry S. Truman

Soapmaking is a unique marriage of science and art. As a science, soap is the chemical combination of fat (either vegetable or animal) and alkali; in home soap production, the alkali used most often is sodium hydroxide, known commonly as lye. The soapmaking process is called *saponification,* meaning "to convert a fat or oil into soap by the action of an alkali."

As an art, it inspires experimentation with colors, textures, scents, and shapes, offering an open invitation to be creative.

Cleansing agents are mentioned in the Bible in Job 9:30, Jeremiah 2:22, and Malachi 3:2. Malachi mentions "the lye of laundrymen." A more specific description of soap is found in the writings of a first-century naturalist-historian, Pliny the Elder, in 77 A.D. Pliny described various forms of hard and soft soaps renowned as *rutilandi capilli,* "making hair shine." These soaps were used by women to cleanse and enhance hair color.

GROWTH OF SOAP INDUSTRY

Ancient history reveals that soap in its early forms was regarded as a mere necessity and was in no way comparable to the giant cosmetic counterpart of today, in either development or commercial popularity. When advancements in the production of soap led to increased public demand and created new markets, the soap industry grew by leaps and bounds. With a heritage steeped in the lavish history of the famous bathhouses of Rome, soap became a valuable article of commerce in early Europe, despite efforts by the early Christian church to discourage bathing as an immodest practice.

In the thirteenth century the soap industry was introduced to France from Italy. At that time most soap was made by boiling goat tallow with beechwood ash (the source of the alkali or lye) and water. Inspired by what they had learned from Italian soapmakers, French soapmakers experimented further to improve soap quality and developed a method of making soap from olive oil instead of animal fats. Around the year 1500 they introduced their discoveries to England, where the industry grew rapidly.

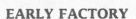

EARLY FACTORY

A remarkably extensive soap factory was found by excavators among the ruins of Pompeii, an ancient city of Italy considered a "resort" area to the Romans.

Colonial American Soap

In the early American colonies, soapmaking was an individual household task as important as spinning, weaving, candlemaking, and other common domestic skills. Hardwood ashes were kept and put into a "leaching barrel," a large wooden barrel with a plugged hole near the base. A thin layer of stones was put in the bottom, and a layer of straw on top of the stones filled up the rest of the barrel. These barrels were kept near the house or barn, where they could catch water runoff from the roof on rainy days. Once the ashes in the leaching barrel were saturated, the plug was removed and the "lye-water" was allowed to drain out into a nonmetal container in the amount needed for a batch of soap. A common test of the lye-water's strength was to dip a feather in it: If the feather dissolved, the lye-water was strong enough to make a batch of soap. If not, the water was poured back into the leaching barrel. These homemade soaps were a soft type that would not be very desirable by today's standards — including a reputation for smelling bad — but they were effective enough for everyday cleaning.

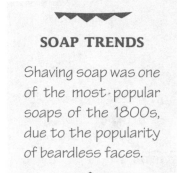

SOAP TRENDS

Shaving soap was one of the most popular soaps of the 1800s, due to the popularity of beardless faces.

In 1621, soap-ash was an important and lucrative export from the colonies to England, providing the colonies with a much-needed source of income. Factory demand in England for both soap-ash and animal fats was enormous. Fifty years later settlements in what is now Maine and New Hampshire gained great wealth from soap-ash and fat exports.

Modernization of Process

The method of acquiring the necessary alkali through wood ashes was tedious, time consuming, and labor intensive. In 1791 Nicolas Leblanc discovered a process for manufacturing caustic soda inexpensively and on a large scale. This revolutionized the industry and eliminated the need to import soap from the colonies. Equally important was new research by the chemist M.E. Chevreul in the 1800s, which clarified the principal differences between fats and oils.

Chevreul's research deciphered the underlying principles of saponification. No discovery has contributed more to the basic, comprehensive understanding of soapmaking.

By the first half of the nineteenth century, both the process and extent of commercial soap production were modernized, and large-scale manufacturing operations developed. It was common for soap to be processed in huge kettles containing from 100,000 to a staggering 1 million pounds of liquid soap. These kettles were heated by open fires and the contents had to be stirred constantly, until the mixture was hand-ladled into large wooden molds, where the saponifying soap hardened until it was ready to be cut.

One of the early American establishments of the soap trade was founded in 1806 by William Colgate of New York. By 1850, New England was the principal center of soap manufacturing in the United States. With the introduction of fancy soaps — perfumed and colored — began soap's unending popularity and variety, leading to the multibillion-dollar soap industry of today.

Commercial soapmaking hardly resembles the simplicity of early production in either ingredients or manufacturing procedures. Most store-bought soaps are now laden with synthetic fillers and additives; and although labeled "pure," soaps are not necessarily wholesome.

WHALE SOAP

Whale oil was used for soapmaking after the process of hydrogenation was invented, which enabled the oil to be hardened to the correct consistency, as well as deodorized.

Use of Milk

Today cosmetic companies include milk in a variety of skin-care-related products. The specific origins of milk-based soaps are not clear, though milk has been used as an ingredient in cosmetics and therapeutic treatments in different cultures for thousands of years. The soothing and moisturizing qualities of milk have made it an increasingly popular ingredient in commercial soaps, especially over the last 30 years.

Because commercial soaps contain additives many of us would like to avoid, however, you may wish to re-create the fundamentals of soapmaking, earning for yourself, as your ancestors did, the deep satisfaction that comes from mastering this ancient art.

A PROFITABLE PURSUIT

In 1622 James I of England granted a monopoly to a soapmaker who was allowed to produce 3,000 tons of soap a year and had to pay the king $100,000 a year for the "privilege." At 4 ounces per bar of soap, that's 24 million bars of soap!

In 1853 a British tax of a penny and a half per pound of soap brought in an annual revenue of more than $5 million.

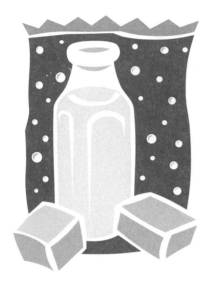

The Fundamentals
of Soapmaking

CHAPTER 2

We learn through experience and no one teaches anyone anything. This is as true for the infant moving from kicking to crawling to walking as it is for the scientist with his equations. If the environment permits it, anyone can learn whatever he chooses to learn; and if the individual permits it, the environment will teach him everything it has to teach.

— Viola Spolin

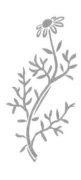

Soapmaking is the chemical combination of fats and alkalis. The process of converting fat or oil into soap by the action of an alkalis is, as I have noted, called saponification. Disregarding all variables, saponification basically boils down to:

Fat + Lye = Soap

Understanding the variables is what allows you to experiment. There are endless varieties that you may wish to explore.

Before beginning there are a few safety practices you must know about. Then we'll take a look at the equipment you will need to make your first batch of soap, with an in-depth discussion of the lye, molds, water, and fats that are critical parts of your soapmaking project. Finally, we'll be ready to go on to our first recipe for basic soapmaking.

Learning successful soapmaking starts with developing excellent and uncompromising safety habits. The alkalis ingredient called for in the soap recipes in this book is sodium hydroxide, commonly known as lye. Sodium hydroxide is a powerful caustic agent that cannot be handled with bare hands, and its fumes must not be inhaled. Companies that manufacture the product warn on their labels that sodium hydroxide burns and is "harmful or fatal if swallowed." Until the fat/lye mixture fully saponifies into soap (approximately 48 hours after being poured into the mold), it will burn the skin.

Working with Lye

Never forget that lye is a powerful and dangerous chemical that must be handled with great care. Everyone who undertakes soapmaking assumes full responsibility for his or her own safety.

Please strictly observe these safe practices:

◆ **Read and observe** the precautionary statements on your lye container.

◆ **Do not undertake soapmaking when tired** or rushed, or while caring for young children. Making soap requires 100 percent undivided attention.

◆ **Always wear safety glasses,** keeping them on from start to finish. Don't risk exposing your precious eyesight to the perils of a lye burn.

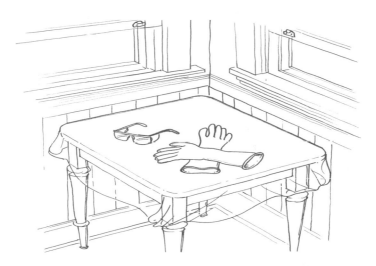

Work in a well-ventilated room, near a window if possible.

- **Always wear rubber gloves.** If you do happen to get any lye on your skin, immediately run cold water on the area.
- **Work in a well-ventilated room, near an open window, preferably.** Do not inhale the fumes. If you live in a region where you must close up the house for the winter, wait for spring!
- **Set aside utensils,** pans, and any other soap-making equipment for soapmaking use only, not to be used later for food preparation.
- **Thoroughly clean** every utensil, container, counter, and tabletop that was used for soap-making immediately after the soap is poured into molds.

BASIC EQUIPMENT AND SUPPLIES

The tools needed to make basic soap are minimal and probably already available in your kitchen. Remember to dedicate your equipment for soapmaking only — do not use it for food preparation. You will need the following:

- 16-ounce (454 g) glass measuring cup
- 2 plastic or stainless-steel spoons
- 2-quart (1.9 l) stainless-steel saucepan
- 8-quart (7.5 l) stainless-steel pot
- Plastic spatula
- Plastic ladle
- Paring knife
- Scale

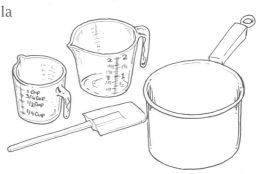

- Plastic wrap and newspaper
- Glass candy thermometer
- Molds (discussed below)
- Spray-on corn oil, mineral oil, or petroleum jelly

Your equipment should primarily be made of glass, stainless steel, or heavy-duty plastic. Never attempt to make soap in aluminum containers — you will ruin both your containers and your batch of soap. Strong plastic spoons are preferable to wood, because the lye will eat away at the wood fibers and eventually ruin the spoon.

You will use the glass measuring cup to measure the water. The spoons and spatula will be needed to stir ingredients and scrape the sides of the pans. You will mix the lye and water in the 2-quart stainless-steel saucepan and melt the fat in the 8-quart stainless-steel saucepan.

Accurate temperature control is a vital part of the saponification process, so a good glass candy thermometer is a must.

Cover your entire working area with either plastic wrap or newspaper to protect work surfaces. Lye is corrosive and can damage areas on which it splashes.

Depending on your type of mold or molds, a good plastic ladle may be necessary to pour small amounts of the liquid soap.

Lye

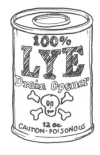

The lye used in the soapmaking process is a chemical called sodium hydroxide. You can purchase sodium hydroxide in your grocery store in 12-ounce (340 g) containers. This is the exact amount needed for the recipes in this book, and it is convenient to have your sodium hydroxide premeasured in a disposable container.

Be absolutely certain that the product you purchase contains only sodium hydroxide. You must read the label, since some brands contain additives that will interfere with the saponification process.

Molds

Before making your soap, you need to consider what your mold or molds will be and prepare them.

The recipes in this book make approximately 8 pounds (3.6 kg) of soap each. If you plan on your bars being 4 ounces (113 g) each, a typical size, you'll get 32 bars of soap per batch.

Molds can be obtained from many sources. Several companies (see suppliers list) specialize in making candy or candle molds that work well as soap molds, giving you a variety of shapes and sizes. Because soap is inclined to absorb color and even corrode as it saponifies, make sure the molds are clear; preferably they will be made of or lined with plastic. However, it may be a bit too expensive to start out buying enough molds for 8 pounds of soap.

An easier, less expensive mold is one made out of wood with dimensions of 20 inches by 14 inches and a depth of at least 2 inches (51 x 36 x 5 cm). If you can find a cardboard or Styrofoam box of this relative size, it will work well also.

Whether made of wood, cardboard, or Styrofoam, you will need to line your mold with plastic, snugging the plastic into the corners, making it as flat as possible on the bottom and sides, and taping it over the edges to hold it in place. Now lubricate the mold

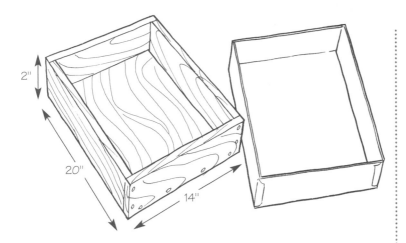

You can make a simple wooden mold (left) or just use a cardboard box (right).

using spray-on corn oil, mineral oil, or petroleum jelly. The spray-on corn oil is the most convenient to use and works the best. Spray a light coating on the bottom and all sides, or use a napkin to rub on a light coating of mineral oil or petroleum jelly.

It is possible to make a grid form to insert into the square mold so the soap will be in forms or bars; this eliminates the need to hand-cut the large block of soap into bars. But you will find that hand-cutting your soap is a very satisfying task; it also results in smoother edges and a better product with much less preparation time.

Water

Using soft water in soapmaking is very important. The mineral deposits found in hard water work against achieving a soap that lathers well. How do you know if you have hard water? Most water, whether it's from a country well or a city waterworks, contains mineral deposits such as lime, iron, sulfur, and more. The amount of mineral deposits always varies with the geographical area but those deposits, no matter how small, will prevent the optimal outcome of your soapmaking. So it is preferable to use water from a water softener, or even rainwater.

If soft water is unavailable, add 1 ounce (28.4 g) of borax to the soap recipe. Borax is a naturally occurring mineral made up of sodium, boron, oxygen, and water. Also called desert salts, it is known to have been used for over 4,000 years. Among other things, it is a famous household cleaning agent. Because of its exceptional water-softening qualities, borax is an excellent soap ingredient that enhances foaming action.

Fats

There are two basic sources of fat for soapmaking: animal and vegetable.

Vegetable oils. Fine cosmetic soaps are often made with a combination of liquid vegetable oils and vegetable shortening. Vegetable shortening usually comes from soybeans. It is economical and readily available at grocery stores. A variety of vegetable oils can be used for soapmaking; each one brings with it its own special qualities. The best and easiest-to-find oils are canola, olive, soy, and corn. As you gain experience and proficiency in soapmaking, the variety of vegetable oils available will offer many avenues for experimentation.

Animal fats. Animal fats have been used in soapmaking since time immemorial. Both pig and beef fat are common, and most soapmakers combine 1 part pork fat with 2 parts beef fat. Before you can use animal fat in soapmaking, it must be rendered. *Rendering* is the process of melting fat and clarifying it, making it free of impurities. You can buy clean rendered lard from your grocer, but it will usually be all pork fat. Soap that is made from all pork fat will be softer and not as white, and it will not last as long as soap made from beef fat. Soap made from all beef fat will be very hard (almost too hard) and nearly white. So it is best when making soap with animal fats to use a combination of both beef and pork.

Do not try to recycle old or used fats such as bacon fat for soapmaking. Although used and even rancid fats will work to make soap, you will lose considerable quality since it is nearly impossible to remove all objectionable odors and get a nice clean color.

If you choose to render your own fat for soapmaking, the time needed for the project will vary according to the amount of fat you render and whether you are using ground fat (ask your butcher to do this for you) or chopped-up chunks. The fat will have to "cook" on *low* heat for 1 to 2 hours, and you cannot leave it unattended.

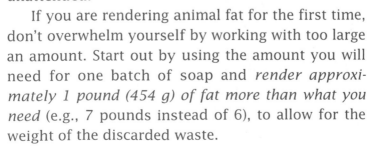

Warning

Use only low heat when rendering fat! It is impossible to rush the rendering process, and attempting to do so only increases the risk of a grease fire.

If you are rendering animal fat for the first time, don't overwhelm yourself by working with too large an amount. Start out by using the amount you will need for one batch of soap and *render approximately 1 pound (454 g) of fat more than what you need* (e.g., 7 pounds instead of 6), to allow for the weight of the discarded waste.

RENDERING ANIMAL FAT

1. Purchase beef and pork fat ground (looking much like very pale hamburger) from your butcher. Fat that is ground up first renders or cooks much faster. If your butcher is unable to grind it for you, cut it into small chunks. Render beef and pork separately.

2. Put each type of fat into a large cooking pot, cover with a lid, and simmer gently over low heat until all of the fat has cooked out and become liquid.

3. Slowly and carefully, pour off the liquid into a clean pot and discard all solids. You may notice a lot of small solids still left, but don't worry: The next step will remove them.

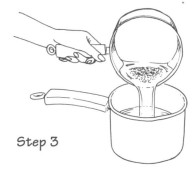

Step 3

4. Allow the fat to cool to 100°F (38°C), measuring with your candy thermometer, and add an equal amount of lukewarm water. The amount does not need to be exactly equal; you can estimate.

5. Bring the fat/water mixture to a gentle simmer and cook, covered, for 15 minutes. Set outside overnight to chill. In the summer months this will have to be done in the refrigerator. In the morning you will find that the fat has risen to the top, and most of the unwanted solids are left in the water.

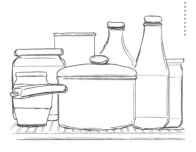

Step 5

6. Using a spatula, remove the top layer of fat. When you lift the hardened fat out of the pan, you may notice a jellylike substance on the bottom. If so, scrape it off and discard it along with the water left in the bottom of the pan.

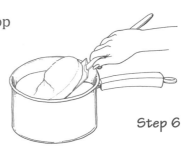

Step 6

7. Place the hardened fat in a clean pan and repeat the process described in Steps 5 and 6, with the following variations. Cut or break fat into chunks, add an equal amount of water and 1 large potato cut in half, cover, and simmer for 15 minutes. Cool overnight, lift the fat out of the water, scrape the bottom clean, and your fat is now properly rendered. The potato helps whiten the fat. If you render large amounts of fat, unused portions can be stored in the freezer for future use.

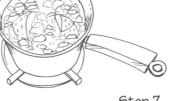

Step 7

PUTTING IT ALL TOGETHER

Now that you have clean, rendered fat, lye, soft water, and a prepared mold or molds . . . let's make soap!

The first time you make a basic soap, you can expect the process to take about 2 hours. After you become proficient, about an hour should suffice, including cleanup, and barring unforeseen chemical complications.

BASIC SOAP RECIPE

32 (4-ounce) bars

6 pounds (2.72 kg) rendered animal fat
(⅔ beef fat + ⅓ pork fat works best)
4½ cups (1.07 l) cold soft water (rainwater or from a water softener)
12 ounces pure lye (available at your
grocery store in this exact size
container)

1. Read and observe the safety recommendations on pages 8–10.

2. Cover all work surfaces with plastic or newspaper. Lay out your soapmaking equipment so that it is at hand, including your molds, prepared as described on pages 12–13. Put on gloves and safety goggles.

3. Heat 4 pounds (1.82 kg) of rendered beef fat and 2 pounds (908 g) of rendered pork fat in the 8-quart stainless-steel pot on low heat. Melt the fats together and hold at 110°F (43°C), measuring with a glass candy thermometer.

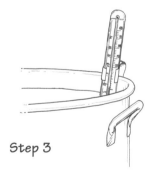

Step 3

4. While the fats are melting slowly (check frequently; stir as needed), measure 4½ cups of cold soft water into the 2-quart stainless-steel saucepan.

5. Working in a well-ventilated area, slowly and carefully add the lye to the water, stirring gently with a plastic or wooden spoon. This mixture will quickly become very hot and may even boil for a few seconds. Do not inhale the fumes — you may want to leave the room for 2 or 3 minutes. Set the mixture aside to cool to 85°F (29°C).

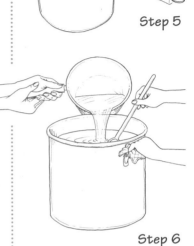

Step 5

6. With the lye/water mixture at 85°F (29°C) and the fat at 110°F (43°C), slowly pour the lye-water into the fat in the larger pot, stirring constantly and gently. Pouring slowly helps the fat and lye-water to blend and reduces the risk of splashing the mixture onto your skin, causing a lye burn.

Step 6

7. Keep stirring this mixture gently as the fat and lye combine. This can take as long as 30 minutes to 1 hour. The mixture will thicken and begin to resemble thin pudding.

Step 8

8. As soon as your spoon starts to feel like it can stand on its own and a few drops of mixture on the surface of the soap leave a distinct pattern, or "trace," pour the mixture into your greased mold(s). The fats and lye are saponifying together; this process will continue for the next 24 to 48 hours.

9. Place the saponifying soap in a draft-free area. Check your soap after 24 hours. It will be ready to cut when it has hardened to the point that you can easily leave a dent in the surface with a firm press of your finger. It must not be too soft, or your cut edges will not be smooth and even. On the other hand, if you wait too long to cut your soap, it will be nearly impossible — the block will have set too hard and become brittle. Soap that has set in the mold for 24 hours is almost always ready to cut. If you feel that it is still too soft after 24 hours, check it every 4 hours. Cut into bars as soon as it is ready.

10. Remove the cut bars of soap from the mold(s) when they are hard enough to remove. It is essential that you allow your new bars of soap to cure for 6 weeks. Then enjoy your first great success! Don't worry about your soap getting too old; the older it gets, the nicer it becomes. Time only enhances soap's character — it never hurts it!

Step 9

Step 10

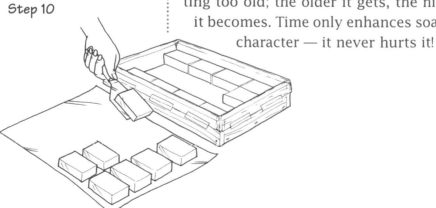

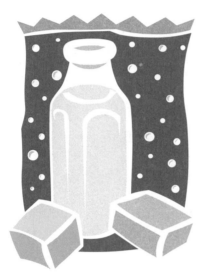

What Is
Milk?

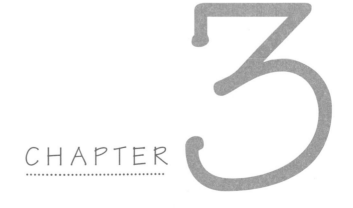

CHAPTER

The cow is of the bovine ilk;
one end is moo, the other, milk.

— Ogden Nash

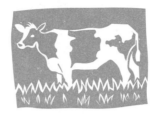

Milk is the fluid secreted by the mammary glands of female mammals. In each species, milk is a complete food for its young. Contrary to Western thinking, milk is not a beverage, it is a food. Milk has been used throughout human history in liquid form, as butter, and as cheese, yogurt, and other fermented products.

When the term *milk* is used in North America, it is generally assumed to refer to cow milk, since most people in the United States and Canada think that milk for human consumption comes only from cows. In fact, buffalo milk is commonly consumed in India, nomadic tribes in arid regions of the Middle East drink horse milk, goat milk is very common in European and Middle Eastern countries, and milk from sheep is used to make excellent cheeses in Europe. Ask a Laplander (a native of northern Sweden, Norway, Finland, or Russia) what she thinks of reindeer milk!

EARLY HISTORY

Animal milk has been used as food since before recorded history. Cheese is mentioned in the Book of Job, and Hindu writings dating to before 1400 B.C. refer to the use of butter as food. It is interesting to note, though, that ancient Greeks, Romans, and Scythians did not use butter as food. They instead applied butter to skin injuries, used the soot of burned butter as an ointment for sore eyes, and most commonly considered pure butter to be an excellent hair dressing.

Before the seventeenth century, *whey* (the watery part of milk that separates from the curd in cheesemaking — it is rich in lactose, minerals, and vitamins) was used as a medicine to treat a variety of ills, including uremia, arthritis, and gout. In the nineteenth century, Europe hosted over 400 whey spas that catered to people seeking healing through whey therapies. From ancient times until today, milk and its by-products have been used not only as excellent sources of nutrition but also for medicinal and cosmetic purposes.

ADULTERATED MILK

Sanitation was almost completely unobserved in early American dairies, and dishonest practices such as diluting milk or adding harmful preservatives such as formaldehyde to it were common.

Before the time of government-regulated dairies, so-called "adulterated" milk was watered down or otherwise tampered with by additions such as chalk, starch, and calf brains.

COMPOSITION OF MILK

But doesn't all milk share the same basic composition? At first you might think so — but the chart on page 24 shows the differences in fat content alone in the milks of different animals.

As you can see, even between animals that appear to be similar to each other, such as the dog and the fox, the donkey and the zebra, and the deer and the goat, milk composition can vary drastically. Even among members of the same species, there will be slight differences in fat content among individual animals, and especially among different breeds of the same animal.

PERCENT OF FAT IN MILK OF VARIOUS ANIMALS

Animal	% fat	Animal	% fat	Animal	% fat
anteater	20.0	elephant	17.6	orangutan	3.5
bison	1.7	fox	5.9	pig	5.1
buffalo	7.9	goat, Nubian	5.0	rabbit	13.1
camel	3.4	goat, Saanen	3.5	rat	12.6
cat	6.3	guinea pig	7.2	reindeer	20.3
cow, Holstein	3.55	hippopotamus	4.5	seal	42.0
cow, Jersey	5.18	horse	1.0	sheep	6.4
deer	19.7	human	3.7	whale	21.2
dog	9.5	llama	3.2	zebra	4.8
dolphin	34.9	monkey	2.7		
donkey	1.4	mule	1.8		

Protein

Milk protein has very high nutritional value for humans and contains all the known and essential amino acids that we cannot synthesize in sufficient quantities to fill our needs. The protein in milk exceeds that of even eggs. Likewise, soap made with milk is naturally protein rich. This unique property of milk-based soap makes it an unequaled favorite for delicate complexions.

PERCENT OF PROTEIN IN MILK

Animal	% protein
cow	3.5
goat	3.5
sheep	5.8
buffalo	3.6
reindeer	10.3

Vitamins

Milk contains vitamin A, converted from carotene by the liver. Carotene affects milk's color — low levels of carotene cause milk to be very white, high levels make milk appear more off-white/creamy yellow in color. Carotene levels themselves fluctuate according to the lactating animal's diet. Animals grazing on lush, springtime green pastures will produce milk that is higher in carotene. Carotene levels play a small role in the subtle color variations of milk-based soaps.

Other vitamins in milk include B_1 (thiamine), B_2 (riboflavin), niacin, B_6 (pyridoxine), pantothenic acid, folic acid, B_{12}, C, and D.

Ash

The percentage of ash in milk reveals the amount of minerals that it contains. Milk ash is literally that: White milk is dried and then burned. The fine, pale powder that remains is called ash. The ash content of goat and cow milk is quite similar: goat, 0.79%; cow, 0.73%.

In the human diet, milk is an important source of minerals. A major source of the important mineral calcium, milk also contains potassium, sodium, magnesium, and phosphorus, plus small amounts of other minerals such as lithium and strontium. Most important to the soapmaker, milk is exposed to high levels of heat when it is combined with lye during the soapmaking process, and ash helps the milk to remain stable under heat.

MILK CHOICES

Cow milk or goat milk? Whole, 2%, or skim? Raw, pasteurized, or powdered? Cream or half-and-half? Homogenized or not? With all these choices, which milk should you use for soapmaking? Let's look at each of these questions in turn.

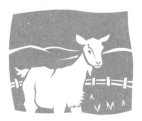

Cow Milk or Goat Milk?

There is no right answer here: It is strictly a matter of personal preference and product availability. Both goat and cow milk make excellent milk soaps. If you live near both a cow and a goat dairy, you have the best of both worlds to experiment in. If you do not have easy access to goat milk and your local grocer does not sell it, your choice has in effect been made for you. Do not linger on the idea that one animal's milk might be better than another's for soapmaking because the truth is that all milks will work in the soapmaking process. More than anything else, the origin of the milk simply determines how distinctive the resulting soap will be.

Whole Milk, 2%, or Skim?

In soapmaking, fat is critical to the saponifying process, so fat content is important. Both cow and goat milk contain similar amounts of fat. Obtain milk of the highest fat content possible for best soap-making results. Do not be tempted to use skim or low-fat milk in soapmaking: Use whole milk.

Raw, Pasteurized, or Powdered?

Pasteurized whole milk purchased from the store will work fine. Where it is available, raw whole milk, fresh from the farm, has one advantage over milk from the store: Raw milk has a higher fat content than commercial milk. It is not unusual to find that the fat content of raw cow milk exceeds 4%.

The standard fat content of commercial whole cow milk available in the dairy section at your local grocery store is standardized at 3% through processing. Milk that is sold as low-fat has 2% fat content, while milk sold as skim has almost no fat at all. Powdered milk does not lend itself to soapmaking because nearly all of the fat has been removed. For the purpose of soapmaking, skim and powdered milk are poor choices and 2% milk would be adequate. Raw (unpasteurized) whole milk, if available, is the best choice, with commercial whole milk a close second choice.

Cream or Half-and-Half?

Can whipping cream, heavy cream, or half-and-half be used in place of whole milk for soapmaking? Yes — the resulting soap is considered *superfatted* because of the higher fat content found in such cream-based milk products. Superfatted refers to soap that has extra emollients incorporated from added oils or moisturizers. When we use cream, the normal proportions of lye to fat are changed, and not all the fat is bound up chemically. Using any type of cream when making milk-based soaps results in a unique, moisturizing cleanser.

When experimenting with using milk creams, substitute an equal amount of cream for either part or all of the milk in a soap recipe. The resulting soap will be very special. Superfatted soaps are a real luxury for the skin!

Homogenized or Not?

Commercial cow milk has been homogenized: The fat globules have been mechanically broken down until they are small enough to remain evenly suspended in the milk. Goat milk is naturally homogenized, because fat globules in goat milk are much smaller than those in cow milk. A very thin cream line may occur in goat milk that has been left to stand undisturbed for 8 or more hours, but most of the cream remains suspended in the milk, so homogenization is unnecessary. Whether the milk is homogenized or not has no effect on its qualities for soapmaking, since homogenization has no effect on fat *content*.

SPEAKING OF MILK

- *Homogenization* is the manufacturing process that forces milk fat to remain evenly distributed throughout the milk instead of rising to the top as cream.
- *Sweetened condensed milk* is milk that has been concentrated to a ratio of 2.2 to 1.0 and contains more than 40 percent sugar!
- *Lactose* is milk sugar.

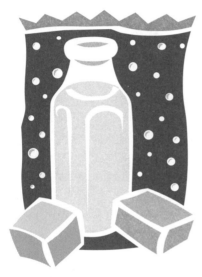

Preparing to Put Milk into Soap

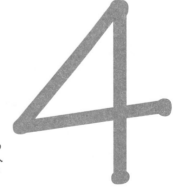

CHAPTER 4

*There is no finer investment for any community
than putting milk into babies.*

— Sir Winston Churchill

Putting milk into babies is a logical practice, but putting milk into soap — can it be done? The answer is a resounding yes. The catch is you have to know the secret to combining the milk and lye.

Many people have attempted to make milk soaps. More often than not they collide with total disaster. Left to their own devices, when the lye and milk are combined they nearly always create a noxious burnt-orange mixture. Then the burnt-orange lye/milk mixture doesn't mix or saponify with the fats or oils. If they mix at all, the defiant mass almost always separates in the mold, leaving lumps of fat floating in orange liquid. Adding insult to injury, proper disposal of this 8 pounds' worth of failure becomes the final frustration.

It is not hard to understand why many people who have experienced such a fruitless result never again rekindle the desire to make milk soap. Failure seems almost inevitable to them and not worth risking a second try. But, to quote Kimberly Ann Walker, "With every failure comes a lesson learned — so the wise saying goes — and a hard lesson learned is a lesson well earned, as everybody knows."

A BEAUTY SECRET REVEALED

To get back into the spirit of things, let's review why anyone would want to try to overcome the noxious lye/milk barrier. Why put milk into soap?

Milk has long been a revered cosmetic ingredient. As part of any beauty regimen, milk has excellent moisturizing qualities and has been heralded throughout the ages as a skin softener even the most delicate skin types can trust. The luxurious milk baths that Cleopatra indulged in to preserve her renowned beauty centuries ago are still remembered today. (I give some sample milk bath recipes in chapter 7 so you can have this same experience!)

In composition, milk is rich in proteins, vitamins, and minerals, nourishing to our bodies both inside and out. In cosmetic use, milk is sometimes referred to as nature's liposomes. Chemically, milk is a *lipoprotein,* one in a class of proteins found in combination with lipids. A *lipid* is an organic substance insoluble in water and usually somewhat greasy to the touch. Lipids, found in most skin creams in the form of wax, animal oil, or vegetable oil, help seal moisture in when applied to the skin, preventing dryness and cracking. Milk is unique in its natural ability to moisturize, nourish, and retain its goodness in your skin — a truly pure, natural beauty aid!

Milk makes a similar contribution to soap, rendering it richer, creamier, and less drying to the skin. Milk is a fragile miracle of nature that cannot be synthetically reproduced. Its gentle properties are easily destroyed by improper handling. It has to be handled with consideration for its delicate nature.

Here's the simple secret to incorporating milk in your soapmaking: All milk for the soapmaking process must be prepared by pasteurizing it, freezing it, and then thawing it when you're ready to make soap.

The results are worth the extra effort they take because milk-based soaps are among the most luxurious soaps you will ever make or use.

PREPARING MILK FOR SOAPMAKING

Two important milk-processing procedures must take place to "prepare" milk properly for being used as a soap ingredient. First, it must be pasteurized. Commercially sold milk has already been pasteurized; raw goat or cow milk purchased fresh from the farm has not been pasteurized, and must be pasteurized at home before it can be used in the soapmaking process.

Second, all milks must be frozen and then thawed before use. Freezing milk increases its stability and makes it less vulnerable to the ravages of the lye when they are mixed together in the soapmaking process.

Pasteurizing and freezing milk. To pasteurize milk, slowly heat it to 155°F (68°C), measuring with a glass candy thermometer. Hold the milk at this temperature for 1 minute, then cover the pan and allow the milk to cool. When cool, pour it into freezable containers (don't use glass), leaving the containers one-quarter empty to allow for expansion. Place in a freezer until frozen solid. The milk can be stored in the freezer for several months. Remove the milk from the freezer to thaw the day before you're ready to make soap. Once it is thawed, the milk will be ready to use.

FROM THE BEGINNING . . . AGAIN!

By now you understand basic soapmaking principles and have perhaps even tried making a batch or two of the basic recipe in chapter 2. If so, you have a general idea of how long it takes to make basic soap. Now that you are ready to make milk soap, plan on spending at least twice that amount of time. It is safe to say that once you become efficient at making milk soap you will need about 1½ hours from start to finish, including cleanup. But for your first few attempts, it would be safest to set aside at least 3 hours.

SPECIAL EQUIPMENT AND SUPPLIES

First you will be adding a few things to your original equipment list, then you will consider the special handling procedures that must be followed when working with milk. By carefully following the simple but specific directions outlined in the next few pages, you will increase your chances of success to almost 100 percent.

Additional Equipment

In addition to the soapmaking equipment described in chapter 2, pages 10 and 11, you will need the following:

- Digital scale to measure liquid vegetable oils
- 3- or 4-quart (3.5 l) stainless-steel pot
- Another 8-quart (7.5 l) stainless-steel pot
- Vinyl window expanders for excellent molds

- Silicone bakery paper for mold liners
- Goat or cow milk — pasteurized, frozen, then thawed
- Large 4-inch (10 cm) putty knife to "screed" the saponifying liquid in the mold
- Small putty knife to cut the soap into bars
- Trisquare — a measuring tool available at your local hardware store
- Eye dropper to measure essential or fragrance oils
- Blender — the secret weapon

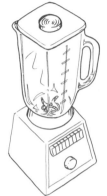

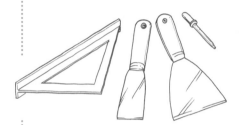

Using Vegetable Oils instead of Animal Fats

A real complement to using milk in making soap is the use of pure vegetable oils in place of animal fats. Vegetable oils associate themselves much better with the concept of being good for the complexion than animal fats do. Their only real drawback is the fact that soap made from vegetable oils doesn't last as long as soap made with animal fats, because animal fat's higher melting point makes soap that is harder at room temperature. But vegetable oils add unique qualities to soap; plus, if you are planning to market your soap, the use of pure vegetable oils also allows you to appeal to consumers who appreciate products honestly labeled "cruelty-free." Many consumers do not have a specific preference for either vegetable oil or animal fat soaps, and — since I have never known anyone to specifically ask for soaps made strictly with animal fats — you automatically appeal to both markets by using pure vegetable oils.

There is a wide variety of vegetable oils to choose from, including solid and liquid forms. *Pure vegetable shortening,* which is made mainly from soybean oil, is very white, nearly odorless, and makes an excellent base. *Olive oil* lends moisturizing qualities and is very mild. Using *extra-light olive oil* reduces its slight odor and contributes to a lighter-colored soap. *Safflower* and *canola oils* add foaming action to soap, helping to create the luxurious lathers we associate with good soap.

All of these oils are very mild to the skin and have very good cleansing qualities. Blending several oils together allows their different strengths to complement one another. I have experimented with many combinations of vegetable oils, and the one I recommend follows.

Ultimately the choice is yours, though, so experiment! You can even try combinations of animal fats and vegetable oils if you'd like a harder soap that lasts longer. Whatever you decide, your soap will be your own creation, reflecting your unique personality.

BASIC VEGETABLE OIL COMBINATION FOR MILK-SOAP RECIPES

3 pounds (1.36 kg) pure vegetable shortening
17 ounces (482 g) extra-light olive oil
12 ounces (341 g) safflower oil
8 ounces (227 g) canola oil

SPECIAL TIPS ON MOLDS AND CURING

Alternative Molds

Milk-based soaps require a bit of extra attention when it comes to selecting and preparing molds. There are several additional pieces of equipment that are useful to have for molding and curing.

Vinyl Window Expanders

For the serious home soapmaker, the best molds to be found for 8-pound batches of soap are *window expanders*. A window expander is a piece of extruded vinyl that is used on the top of vinyl windows as a gap filler during installation. Window expanders are made in white and brown, but only white should be used for molds, because saponifying soap will often absorb color. Expanders can be purchased from most vinyl window manufacturers and usually come in 16-foot lengths. The interior measurements of 1½ inches high and 3¼ inches wide make perfect dimensions for strips of single bars. These will give you soap strips that can easily be sliced into bars before removing from the mold.

To customize the mold to fit the recipe in this chapter, cut the expander into lengths of 69⅞ inches.

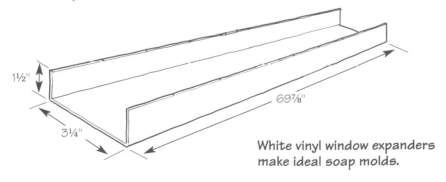

1½"   3¼"   69⅞"

White vinyl window expanders make ideal soap molds.

Seal the ends with a piece of taped PVC or vinyl, or duct tape (see illustration at right). Then measure and mark the upper edge of the frame every 2¼ inches with an indelible marker. These are your cutting marks. Each mold will contain 31 bars weighing approximately 4.2 ounces before curing.

Lining the mold. Milk-based soaps tend to stick to molds much more than other soaps do. To eliminate this problem almost entirely, I recommend lining your molds with silicone bakery paper. This is a tough Teflon-type paper used in bakeries as a cake-pan liner and can usually be purchased there in small amounts. Bakeries reuse their paper several times, but you will get only one use out of it. The saponifying soap ruins it. For the one time it does its job, though, it is worth it.

For each 69⅞-inch expander strip, you will need one sheet of silicone bakery paper cut into three pieces and folded as shown in the illustration below. Cover the mold ends with plastic

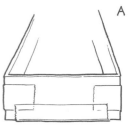

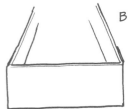

Seal the end by taping a piece of PVC over it (A), or with a strip of duct tape (B).

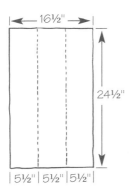

Cut the full sheet of bakery paper into thirds (dotted lines are cutting lines).

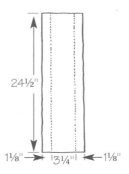

Fold each third of the bakery paper along the dotted lines. Measurements are approximate.

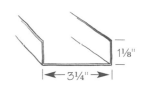

One sheet of cut and folded bakery paper is enough to line one 69⅞" mold with overlap between sheets.

packing tape before lubricating to ensure a good seal. Set the bakery paper into your mold and lubricate with spray-on corn oil or mineral oil.

When pouring the soap into this mold, make sure to hold the bakery paper down with a knife until the soap flows over it and weighs it down, to prevent seepage under the paper. Once the mold is full, if needed, you can use the cement technique known as screeding to even out the surface of the liquid. Pull the flat edge of a large putty knife or spatula across the entire surface of the mold, from one end to the other. This reduces lumps and other irregularities, making the surface of the liquid soap nice and smooth.

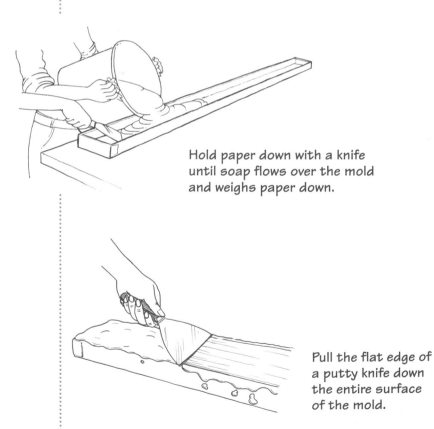

Hold paper down with a knife until soap flows over the mold and weighs paper down.

Pull the flat edge of a putty knife down the entire surface of the mold.

Cutting bars. As mentioned on page 20, it is important that you cut your soap after 24 hours to get the cleanest edges. To cut the bars in this mold, use a trisquare. Set it parallel to each 2¼-inch mark to guide a straight cut, then slice each bar straight down with a narrow blade putty knife, sliding it from one side of the mold to the other. Cut the entire strip of bars first, then remove one bar and decide whether the bars are hard enough to remove or whether they need to sit another few hours before removing all of them.

Use a trisquare to mark the spot, then cut cleanly from side to side with a putty knife.

PVC Plumbing Pipe

Another good mold source is a 1-foot length of round 2-inch PVC plumbing pipe with a removable cap on one end. You will need 5 or 6 of these pipes for most recipes in this book. Pour the soap into the pipe. When it is hardened, you can remove the cap, push the soap out, and slice it into rounds. To make the removal easier, apply mineral oil liberally to the inside of the pipe before adding soap. These round slices make excellent little shaving soaps that fit nicely into shaving mugs.

Slice soap into rounds as you push it through pipe.

Loofah Sponge Soap Scrubs

Here's a way to create exotic soaps and scrubs:

1. Slice natural loofah sponges into 2-inch (5 cm) pieces.

2. Wrap the outside of each loofah piece in waxed paper, and set them on end on another piece of waxed paper.

3. Fill the hollow insides with soap.

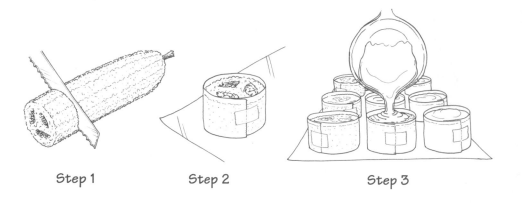

Step 1   Step 2   Step 3

Allow these soap-filled loofahs to cure for 6 weeks and what a wonderful gift idea you'll have — not to mention another very marketable soap item!

Curing and Drying Soap

Drying racks. Once the cut soaps are removed from the mold, they will need to cure for 6 weeks. Large plastic bread racks work great for this purpose. The bottoms are meshed to allow for good air circulation, and they can be stacked on top of each other to maximize use of space. If you stand the soap bars up on the narrow ends, each bread rack will hold three batches or 93 bars of soap (my racks measure 26½" x 22".

Discarded bread racks no longer in good enough condition to be used for shipping bread can often be obtained from bread companies by special request. Whatever your choice of drying rack, make sure it's plastic. Avoid wood, aluminum, steel, and galvanized steel, as none of these materials will retain its integrity under the soap's caustic curing. Wood will absorb moisture from the soap and start to bleed stain into the soap. Contact with aluminum and galvanized steel could turn the soap black, and steel will start to corrode before the soap is cured.

Cure soap on a plastic rack.

Curing environment. The 6-week curing process should take place in a cool but dry area, and the bars should be lightly covered with a sheet of plastic wrap to protect them from dust. If the room is too humid, the bars will not cure well. If a dehumidifier is available, it will expedite the curing process and ensure more thorough curing. Be aware that as soap cures, it shrinks; you will notice as much as a 16 percent decrease in each bar's original weight by the time it has fully cured.

ADDITIONAL SOAP INGREDIENTS

The most exciting part of learning how to make milk soap is that once you've gotten the knack of it, you can expand on the basic recipe and explore variations. There are many natural ingredients that you can put into milk soap to enrich its qualities. These natural extras appeal to different skin types and personalities. Once you master the basic milk-based soap recipe in chapter 5, you may want to experiment with adding other ingredients. Following are a few to try.

Herbs. Herbs are a wonderful addition to milk-based soap. You can use them fresh or dried. Herbs such as lavender, chamomile, rose petals, and rosemary each add a distinct identity and evoke different associations. These herbs will not keep their original colors, since most of these colors will fade in reaction to the lye, but their aromas and textures will be subtly captured.

Exfoliators. A number of ingredients add exfoliating qualities to soap, which gently scrape away dead skin cells and let the new ones underneath shine and breath.

Oatmeal. Oatmeal soap has been an enduring favorite for generations. The addition of ground oatmeal to soap gives it a rich texture that favors normal, oily, and dry skin types. Soap containing ground oatmeal will have a lovely ivory/tan color.

Cornmeal. Cornmeal imparts a golden yellow cast and pleasant, naturally sweet fragrance to each bar. It gives soap a strong, but not harsh, cleansing property that makes it a perfect all-purpose hand soap.

Bran. Bran contributes a special aesthetic trait to soap, in addition to its mild exfoliating qualities. Bars containing bran are a pale ivory color with a spackling of warm brown flecks throughout.

Almond meal. Ground almonds help create a gentle cleansing bar that gently exfoliates and moisturizes for dry skin types.

Eggshells. This is a soap ingredient that has powerful cleansing abilities as a hand soap. It is not recommended as an ingredient for face soap because it is too abrasive. The addition of ground eggshells will make a strong soap that will be more than a match for stubborn dirt on hands or feet.

Lanolin. This is the grease or fat that comes from sheep's wool. It is used in cosmetics as a neutral, nonirritating base for ointments and creams because of its excellent moisturizing qualities. You may know that sheep shearers rarely suffer from dry, chapped hands; they have a reputation for having the softest hands anywhere! It is a perk from handling so much lanolin-rich wool.

If you are familiar with lanolin, you know it is very thick and tacky, dark yellowish in color, and has a very strong sheep odor. Do not let its outward appearance and smell fool you into thinking it will not work well in soap. Lanolin may have a bit of an odor, but it does not stand out once the soap is made. It is an excellent soap ingredient that will make some of your best moisturizing soap.

You should only use pure *nonhydrous* lanolin — that is, lanolin that has never had water or other ingredients whipped into it to make it creamy. Your pharmacist will carry it in 1-pound (454 g) quantities.

Honey. For the same reasons that honey is used as a facial pack and an ingredient in hand lotions, it can also be a soothing soap ingredient. Honey is a source of vitamins, minerals, and amino acids, and even has slight antiseptic properties. It is an especially good ingredient for delicate skin.

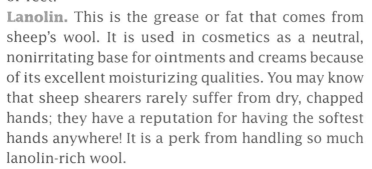

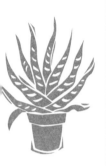

Cocoa butter. This is pure cocoa fat extracted from ground and crushed cocoa beans. Cocoa butter is considered to be nourishing as well as moisturizing for the skin. Try adding it to the milk-based soap recipe along with vanilla, coconut, and almond fragrance for an irresistible soap!

Aloe vera. Famous for its healing qualities, aloe vera comes from the plant of the same name. The gel-like substance that is extracted from the plant lends its gentle nature to produce a mild, all-purpose soap that is soothing to the skin.

Colors and fragrances. Soap can be enhanced by natural colors and fragrances, but both can be difficult to use for the same reason: Because of its caustic nature, the saponifying liquid that will soon become soap burns out both color and fragrance derived from natural sources. Natural fragrances and colors are much more delicate than their synthetic counterparts, so you cannot expect to create the strong colors and heavy scents that you find in

PRESERVATIVES

As a rule, homemade soap does not need preservatives to protect it from becoming stale or rancid. As it ages, all soap just becomes a more effective cleaning agent. Correctly made, the soap recipes in this book have no time limit on the curing process, so you do not need to worry abut it having a shelf life that must be prolonged by preservatives. Time will not cause this milk-based soap to become rancid — time will only cause it to become better soap! However, don't forget that soap is best enjoyed when used.

store-bought soaps. Instead, you will be delighted with the subtle hints of color and essence that can be extracted from nature's pantry. In any case, color and smell do not make soap work better — even if they do make it more distinguished.

Colors from Nature

The basic color variations you can expect to get from natural sources are pale green from rosemary, light brown from cinnamon and cloves, pale yellow from cornmeal, and varying shades of creams and tans from the rest.

Adding chopped herbs or plant material such as rose petals, lavender, and mints — or adding ground grains such as oatmeal, cornmeal, and almond meal — will also add a pretty speckled look and a bit more texture to your soap.

Synthetic perfumes and colors offer a wide array of choices but lack the character, charm, and goodness of natural products. Candlemaking supply companies offer dyes that hold up fairly well in the saponifying process (they can also be a source for molds for your soaps). Herbal supply companies often offer not only essential oils but realistic-smelling fragrance oils as well, both of which you might find better suited for your soap. You'll find addresses for some of these companies at the end of the book.

Achieving colors and fragrances from natural sources sometimes goes hand in hand with adding specialty ingredients to the soap. For example, adding cornmeal will make the soap slightly yellowish with a sweet corn smell. Cinnamon will give you a brownish soap that smells like the spice.

Selecting Scents

The following list includes scents that are strong enough to withstand the saponifying process. These can also be mixed and matched to create unique fragrances.

Almond	Orange
Cinnamon	Patchouli
Citronella	Peach
Cloves	Pennyroyal
Eucalyptus	Peppermint
Jasmine	Rose
Lavender	Rosemary
Lemon	Sage
Musk	Vanilla

FRAGRANCE TERMS

Essential oils are highly concentrated extracts derived from the leaves, berries, flowers, petals, twigs, bark, or stem of plants through a specialized distillation or expression process. These oils usually bear the scent or fragrance of the original plant. The prices vary and can be quite high, depending on the particular plant (some are more difficult to produce than others). But a little bit goes a long way. Essential oils are also believed to have therapeutic properties.

Fragrance oils are synthetically produced imitations of plant essences. They are far less expensive than essential oils and are less vulnerable to spoilage. The best way to select fragrance oils is to smell enough until you find one you like.

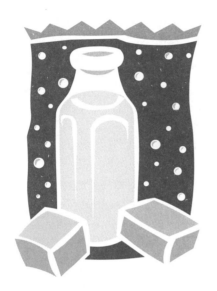

The Standard
Milk-Based
Soap Method

CHAPTER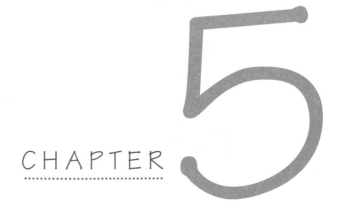

TRUE creativity often starts where language ends.
— Arthur Koestler

Adding milk to the soapmaking equation is a challenge, and using the proper technique is critical to success. There are so many variables to consider, each one claiming a rightful place in the procedure. Let's review the things that will make the most difference in producing a quality batch of soap.

Be Patient

Foremost, resist the temptation to rush. Soapmaking is a process that cannot be hurried. This is especially true with milk soap. Every batch will be slightly different even if you follow the recipe exactly every time. Allow for each batch to develop its individual character in its own time. Becoming impatient will only waste the time you already have invested.

Take Careful Notes

You do not learn to make soap by reading a book, even this one! Books can only offer guidelines based on the author's experience. The more you make soap, the more the soap will be able to teach you how to make it better. Take notes. Document every detail of each batch right down to the weather that day and include the date. This running record will allow you to refer back and evaluate your procedures after the soap has cured and you decide what you do and don't like about it. You can also keep track of your progress as a soapmaker; years down the road you will feel deep satisfaction for all you have learned.

Use Quality Ingredients

As with so many things in life, your soap will only be as good as the ingredients you put into it. Do not lessen the quality of your soap by cutting corners to save a few pennies. Soap that is not as lathery, long lasting, nice smelling, and even colored as it should be will make the time and money you have invested not worth the bother. Whether your soap is destined to be a product you market or a gift for family and friends, take pride in your work. The fine quality you achieve will be a credit to you as a soapmaker and will contribute to the good reputation of all hand-made soaps!

Choose and Prepare Milk Carefully

Although milk from any animal can be used for making soap, the two most common and available milks on the market are cow and goat milk. Goat milk is naturally homogenized: Its milk fat does not separate or rise to the top as cow milk's does. Left to stand for a day or two, goat milk forms only a thin cream on its surface. Cow milk is mechanically homogenized, so most people today have rarely seen cow milk with a natural layer of cream on the surface. Consequently, most of us have been conditioned by our over-processed society to consider a cream line on our milk a defect or just plain undesirable.

Both milks have about the same percentage of butterfat, with an average range of 2.5 to 4.0 percent, but goat milk is preferable because of its natural homogenization. It has smaller fat globules than cow milk, and its fat content tends to mix better and saponify more readily. In addition, goat milk enjoys a justified reputation for being unique and healthful. If you don't own goats, raw goat milk can be purchased from dairy goat breeders (see resource list).

Preparing goat milk for soapmaking. Goat milk must first be pasteurized by slowly heating it to 155°F (68°C). Then it should be cooled, poured into freezable containers (don't use glass; leave container one-quarter empty to allow for expansion). Whatever kind of milk you select (see pages 26 to 28), it must be frozen before use in soapmaking. Freezing the milk causes it to become more stable in the soapmaking process and less likely to succumb to the ravages of the lye when they are mixed together (see page 32 for instructions).

Measure Accurately

Soapmaking is an exacting chemical science. You are setting in motion molecular changes with the goal of achieving a specific outcome. For best results, measure as precisely as possible. This means measuring by weight, not volume. A good digital scale affords accurate control of the compounds you are working with, and your records will be a more detailed and dependable resource.

Work with a Partner

Because more quality control and specific procedures are required to make milk soap than other kinds, I recommend working with a partner. There will be points throughout the process where you will wish you had four hands, so enlist the help of a friend or relative. A second person can also increase the safety factor and decrease the margin of error.

TIPS FOR A SAFE WORK ENVIRONMENT

There are important considerations for the work environment that need to be established before soapmaking can safely begin. Soapmaking will take your undivided attention from start to finish, so allow yourself plenty of time free from distractions, phone calls, and other interruptions.

- **Stable work surface.** The work surface should be a roomy, stable area such as a cleared kitchen countertop. Avoid rickety tables.
- **Cover work surface.** All work surfaces should be covered with newspaper or plastic to protect them from accidental splashes or spills.
- **Proper ventilation.** Make soap in a well-ventilated room, preferably at a time of year when the windows can be left open. Avoid breathing fumes from the lye-milk mixture. Plan to leave the room immediately for a couple of minutes when the milk and lye are first mixed if the fumes become too strong.
- **Children.** Young children should be safely supervised away from the soapmaking work area. Older children may observe the soapmaking process from a safe distance, though they should leave the room when the milk and lye are first mixed because of the fumes. Rubber gloves and safety glasses are a must for their protection.
- **Accessible tools and equipment.** Lay out and organize your soapmaking equipment so it is easily within reach. Once you start to mix the ingredients, it will be too late to stop and hunt for things.
- **Safety glasses and gloves.** Wear safety glasses and rubber gloves throughout the soapmaking process. Practice good safety habits!

MILK MEETS LYE MAKING SOAP

Well-made milk soap is created with the maximum amount of milk that can be included in proportion to the lye and fat used per batch, not just a smattering of the ingredient to justify saying it's in there. If milk is going to be expected to perform as an active ingredient, then it has to exist in each bar in a substantial amount. Ideally each 4-ounce bar should be able to claim 1.5 to 2 ounces of its weight in milk.

Understanding the basic recipe. This standard recipe uses the combination of vegetable oils recommended on page 53.

No matter what additional ingredients you choose to add — fragrance, herbs, grains — this basic recipe will serve as your starting point. This recipe applies the soapmaking technique detailed in chapter 2 to making milk soap, anticipating potential obstacles. I encourage you to follow this basic recipe for making several batches to start. Then, in chapter 6, we'll look at many of the variations to this basic recipe that you may want to try.

As you will see, the biggest challenge is putting the lye into 3 pounds of milk. That is a large volume of a fluid that doesn't hold up well to being combined with a caustic chemical.

Dismiss for good the notion that you can pour lye into milk with the same ease that you would when making soap with water! It can certainly be done, but if you want the milk to work for you in the soapmaking process, you will have to work with it and within its tolerance for being chemically processed and altered.

BASIC RECIPE FOR MILK-BASED SOAP

32 (4-ounce) bars

3 pounds (1.36 kg) pure vegetable shortening

17 ounces (482 g) extra-light olive oil

12 ounces (341 g) safflower oil

8 ounces (227 g) canola oil

3 pounds (1.36 kg, or approximately 6 cups)
goat or cow milk, prepared for soapmaking
(see page 32)

12 ounces (312 g) pure sodium hydroxide (lye)

1 ounce (28.4 g) borax

½ ounce (14.2 g) white sugar

½ ounce (14.2 g) glycerine

1. Begin by observing the safety recommendations in chapter 2, "Safety First." Cover all work surfaces with plastic or newspaper, prepare your mold(s) (see pages 12–13), and lay out your soapmaking equipment so it is within reach. See pages 33–34 for a complete list of what you'll need. Once you start to mix ingredients, it will be too late to stop and hunt for things. Wear safety glasses and rubber gloves at all times in this process. Soapmaking will take your undivided attention from start to finish, so allow yourself plenty of time free from distractions to complete the task.

2. Melt the vegetable shortening in an 8-quart pot over low heat on the stove.

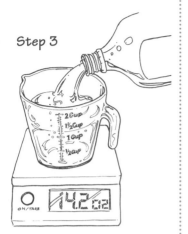

Step 3

3. Weigh the liquid oils carefully on a digital scale; add them to the pan with the shortening. Heat the combined ingredients only until the vegetable shortening is completely melted, then immediately remove from heat. Do not overheat your oils — it is possible to ruin them for soapmaking by overheating or scorching them. You are not deep-frying french fries, you are making soap. Set aside until step 9.

4. Fill your sink with cold water. Add 4 to 6 trays of ice cubes to the water.

5. Put the 3 pounds of cold milk, pre-pared as recommended for soapmaking (see page 32), into a 3- or 4-quart stain-less-steel pot. Carefully place the saucepan into the ice water. Stabilize the floating pan by placing several plas-tic cups filled with water around it.

Step 5

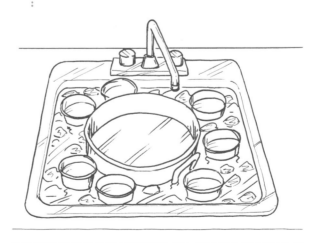

6. Making sure you have gloves on, measure 12 ounces of lye into a 16-ounce glass measuring cup, using the digital scale for accuracy.

7. Now **very** slowly pour the lye into the cold milk in the ice-water bath, stirring all the while with a heavy-duty plastic spoon. This pouring process should take *no less* than 15 minutes. This slow introduction of the lye into the milk, in combination with the cold bath, prevents the lye from achieving the extreme temperatures and aggressive caustic action that would otherwise scorch the milk into a useless burnt-orange mess. This is one of the most important keys to success. You are taming lye's hostile nature by forcing it to stay cool. By doing so, you are protecting the milk from damage. Although cool from being in the cold bath, the milk/lye mixture is, nevertheless, still extremely corrosive, and you must avoid letting it contact your bare skin.

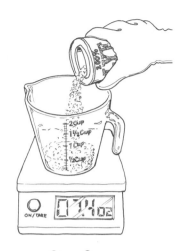

Step 6

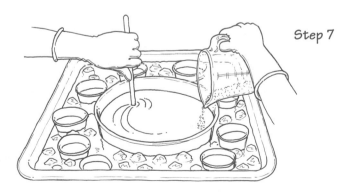

Step 7

8. It is important now to gauge the temperature of the lye/milk mixture so that it does not drop below 80°F (27°C). You want to keep the mixture cool enough to prevent the milk from scorching, but warm enough to prevent the milk and lye from saponifying. Saponification occurs between the milk and the lye at this temperature because there is enough fat in milk to cause this action. The two main mistakes you might make at this point are allowing the lye/milk mixture to get too cool, and letting it sit too long before combining it with the oils. Both of these scenarios could cause the mixture to congeal into a noxious and useless custard-textured mass that would need to be scooped out of the pan instead of poured. So guard the temperature and keep stirring. Keep the temperature of the mixture right at 80°F (27°C), and remove it from the cold-water bath as soon as the lye and milk are combined. You will notice that the milk turns a bright yellowish color once the lye has been combined with it if the process has been successful.

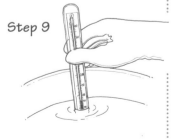

Step 9

9. Over low heat, reheat the oils to a temperature of 125°F (52°C). Remove from heat. Be careful not to overheat or scorch the oils.

10. Slowly pour the lye/milk mixture into the oil. Add the borax, sugar, and glycerin. Stir constantly, being careful not to splash any on your skin. The entire mass will get very warm; just keep stirring gently. You will probably notice the lye/milk mixture refusing to join itself with the oils, even sinking to the bottom of the pan, if you stop stirring. Be patient.

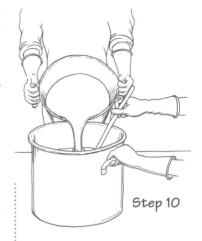

Step 10

11. The blender is an invaluable tool for making milk-based soap from this point on, until the saponifying mixture is poured into the mold. It is the mechanism that forces the lye/milk mixture and the oils to join together and begin to saponify into a smooth, even-textured soap.

Use a plastic ladle to scoop evenly mixed amounts of the oil/lye mixture from the pan into the blender. Fill the blender halfway. **Secure the lid onto the blender carefully before switching it on!** Run the blender for 1 minute on medium speed, remembering to keep stirring the contents of the pan in the sink in the meantime. You will notice the liquid in the blender becoming a lovely pale cream color.

Step 11

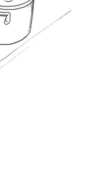

After 1 minute, pour the contents of the blender into the second 8-quart saucepan. Now you have two pans to stir and a blender to run — so you can appreciate why a partner is so helpful! Repeat this entire procedure until all of the original mixture of oils and lye/milk has been blended.

12. Quickly wash out the first saucepan (which is now empty), dry it well, and repeat the whole process, going from the second pan to the blender for 1 minute and then to the first pan, stirring both pans all the while. It is during the second blending that you can add fragrance or specialty ingredients such as herbs or grains (see chapter 6 for recipe suggestions). You will now see little or no separation of the oils from the rest of the mixture; after the second blending the liquid mass will be ready to pour. It will have thickened up somewhat, but even if it seems a little thin, it will still be ready for the mold. If it really seems too thin, you can repeat the blending procedure a third time.

Step 12

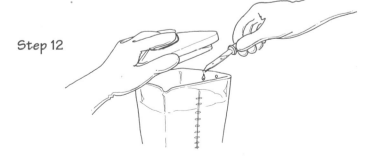

13. Pour the mixture into the prepared mold and screed the top surface (see pages 37–38 for mold preparation and screeding technique).

14. Allow the saponifying liquid to sit uncovered and undisturbed in a draft-free area. Do *not* cover it so as to allow unnecessary moisture to escape. The air humidity will have an effect on this part of the process, and it is better for the mold to be in an area of low humidity. After 12 hours have passed you may notice that sweatlike beads of tan-colored moisture have come to the surface. This occurs occasionally and is nothing to be alarmed about. The beads will normally evaporate on their own after 24 hours. You can gently wipe off those that don't with a paper towel before cutting the bars.

15. Cut into bars after 24 hours, then allow the cut soap to remain in the mold for another 24 hours, until it is hard enough to hold its shape when removed from the mold. If it is too soft, check it every 4 hours until it is ready. Do not wait over 24 hours to cut, or the soap will become too brittle. See pages 20 and 39 for cutting instructions.

16. Allow the bars to cure for 6 weeks in a dry, cool room. Cover lightly with plastic wrap to protect from dust.

No matter how careful you are, problems may still present themselves and you will need to figure out what went wrong and how to avoid similar situations in the future. Working with a fragile substance such as milk and a highly corrosive substance such as lye, and expecting the two to bond perfectly with each other and the oils every time, is unrealistic. Plus, you further complicate the chemistry of the saponification process when you introduce herbs, grains, fragrances, or any other ingredient to the mixture.

Learning the art of soapmaking means learning to discern when the problems you encounter have reasonable and workable solutions and when they don't. Be aware that some problems will simply remain mysteries. In these cases you may have to dispose of a batch that has turned into a mess.

APPRECIATE YOUR FIRST EFFORTS

Your first bars of milk-based soap will be a real treasure, an accomplishment you can be proud of. You will find its rich, creamy lather and silky texture a true reward for your patience and perseverance. Yes, your first few batches may present glitches that might challenge your resolve to master the technique of making milk soap — but practice and endurance will pay off. You now have the keys to success, all you have to do is unlock the door!

Failure to Saponify

It happens to the best of soapmakers once in a while, when a batch of liquid soap refuses to make the chemical changes needed to saponify, especially when you are working with milk.

When you hit a stubborn batch that seems to refuse to set up, starting over is really your best choice. Usually, if you have to do too much to the mixture to try to fix it, the mixture would not have turned out good soap anyway. Let's take a look at problems that can arise and how to overcome them when possible.

Combining the Milk and Lye

Review the recommended guidelines for milk preparation and handling in chapter 4 (page 32) before adding the lye to it. This is your best defense against potential problems. Even so, remember that milk is a natural product with a range of naturally occurring variations and on rare occasions the milk may just refuse to mix properly with the lye. The mixture might become overheated and turn a burnt-orange color, and the milk fat may float to the top. If this occurs, the only thing you can do is dispose of it and start over. If you press on and use it anyway, the burned milk will only cause problems later in the process. It will not saponify well with the oils and the final color and quality of your soap will be very unsatisfactory.

A less frustrating problem with the milk/lye mixture may arise if you allow it to cool too much or sit too long before combining it with the oils. The mixture will become custardlike and will have to be scooped out of the pan. You can still add it to the oils, though; usually the blender will mix it well enough that it will not pose any problems to the final results. The milk/lye mixture will be more stable to work with if you maintain the temperature so it can be poured out of the pan.

Separation of Fats/Oils from Lye Mixture

Correct saponifying action is when the fats/oils combine with the lye to become soap. Sometimes the chemical process of saponification will go awry, and separation will occur after you've poured the mixture into the mold(s).

You can expect the oils and the lye mixture not to blend together easily when you first combine them; that is why the blender is so important. The blender forces the oils and lye mixture to join and mechanically prevents separation as long as the mixture is being blended. By the time you pour the contents of the blender into the pan, most of the separation problem has been worked out.

Once in a while, though, separation will occur after the liquid mixture has been poured into the mold(s). If this happens, consider the batch ruined and discard the whole thing. You might be tempted to pour the mass back into the saucepan and reheat it to encourage saponification. **This is extremely dangerous,** and futile in any case. The liquid is highly corrosive and lye is very sensitive to being heated. The goal of the soapmaking process has been to temper lye's hot nature; in heating it, you would be encouraging the lye to become chemically aggressive, and you'll ultimately lose control over the process.

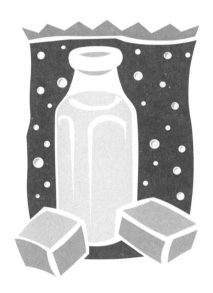

Specialty

Recipes

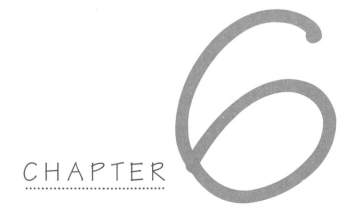

CHAPTER 6

"Science" means simply the aggregate of all the recipes that are always successful.

—Paul Valéry

Once you've made several batches of soap using the method described in chapter 5, you'll have a solid foundation for understanding the technique of making milk-based soaps. Let's expand on the theme by exploring specialty recipes that introduce a unique character into each batch of soap. The possibilities are open-ended. Try these, and then experiment with creating your own.

Before You Begin: Important Reminders

Before you start making any of the recipes in this chapter, observe the safety recommendations in chapter 2, "Safety First."

RECIPE INSTRUCTIONS

All the recipes in this chapter follow the steps for making milk soap on pages 53–59. Note any special instructions included for the particular recipe.

HONEY CREAM
32 (4-ounce) bars

~~~~~~

This is a mild, fragrance-free soap made with goat milk, goat cream, and honey. It is especially gentle and good for delicate skin types. Many people enjoy using this soap on children because of its mildness. Goat cream makes this soap extra rich. It can be obtained by running the milk through a cream separator. If a cream separator is not available, it is nearly impossible to obtain cream from the whole milk, because goat milk is naturally homogenized. Substitute cow cream.

Prepare by covering all work surfaces with plastic or newspaper. Lay out your soapmaking equipment so it is within reach. Wear safety glasses and gloves. Have your mold(s) prepared.

3   pounds (1.36 kg) pure vegetable shortening
17 ounces (482 g) extra-light olive oil
12 ounces (341 g) safflower oil
8   ounces (227 g) canola oil
1   pound (454 g, or approximately 2 cups) goat or cow cream, prepared as the milk was for soapmaking
2   pounds (908 g, or approximately 4 cups) goat or cow milk, prepared for soapmaking
12 ounces (340 g) pure sodium hydroxide (lye)
1   ounce (28.4 g) borax
¼ ounce (7.1 g) honey
¼ ounce (7.1 g) glycerin

Special instruction. Add the cream to the milk before combining the milk with the oils.

OATMEAL SOAP
32 (4-ounce) bars

〰〰〰

Oatmeal makes this recipe just right for oily complexions. It is deliciously scented with vanilla and almond fragrance oils.

3	pounds (1.36 kg) pure vegetable shortening
17	ounces (482 g) extra-light olive oil
12	ounces (341 g) safflower oil
8	ounces (227 g) canola oil
3	pounds (1.36 kg, or approximately 6 cups) goat or cow milk, prepared for soapmaking
12	ounces (340 g) pure sodium hydroxide (lye)
1	ounce (28.4 g) borax
¼	ounce (7.1 g) white sugar
¼	ounce (7.1 g) glycerin
½	cup (118 ml) rolled oats
¼	ounce (7.1 g) almond fragrance oil
¼	ounce (7.1 g) vanilla fragrance oil

Special instructions. Prepare the oatmeal by putting ½ cup of rolled oats in the blender and grating it for 60 seconds, or until you get a medium-coarse powder. Refining the oatmeal in this manner helps it to better blend into the soap, and creates a more finely textured soap. Add the oatmeal when you run the liquid mixture through the blender for the first time, and add the fragrance oils when you run the liquid mixture through the blender for the second time.

SHEPHERD'S PRIDE
32 (4-ounce) bars

～～～～

This soap is enriched with pure lanolin and aloe vera, both renowned for their healing and moisturizing qualities. It is scented with jasmine and is excellent for dry skin.

3 pounds (1.36 kg) pure vegetable shortening
17 ounces (482 g) extra-light olive oil
12 ounces (341 g) safflower oil
4 ounces (113 g) canola oil
4 ounces (113 g) lanolin
3 pounds (1.36 kg, or approximately 6 cups) goat or cow milk, prepared for soapmaking
12 ounces (340 g) pure sodium hydroxide (lye)
1 ounce (28.4 g) borax
¼ ounce (7.1 g) white sugar
¼ ounce (7.1 g) glycerin
½ ounce (14.2 g) aloe vera
½ ounce (14.2 g) jasmine fragrance oil

Special instructions. Melt the lanolin with the oils. Add the fragrance oil and aloe vera when you run the liquid mixture through the blender for the second time.

ALMOND-JOY
32 (4-ounce) bars

〰〰〰

Sweet almond oil, ground almonds, and almond fragrance create a wonderful soap that works well for dry skin.

 3 pounds (1.36 kg) pure vegetable shortening
17 ounces (482 g) extra-light olive oil
20 ounces (568 g) sweet almond oil
 3 pounds (1.36 kg, or approximately 6 cups) goat or cow milk, prepared for soapmaking
12 ounces (340 g) pure sodium hydroxide (lye)
 1 ounce (28.4 g) borax
¼ ounce (7.1 g) white sugar
¼ ounce (7.1 g) glycerin
½ cup (118 m) raw almonds
½ ounce (14.2 g) almond fragrance oil

Special instructions. Combine the almond oil with the other oils at the beginning of the process. Grate ½ cup of raw almonds in the blender for 60 seconds, or until you get a coarse powder. Add this almond meal to the liquid mixture when it's run through the blender for the first time. Add the fragrance oil when you run the liquid mixture through the blender for the second time.

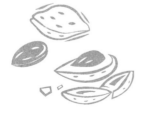

PEACHES AND CREAM
32 (4-ounce) bars

This is a lovely, very popular soap made with goat cream and peach fragrance. Goat cream makes this soap rich and creamy and can be obtained by running the milk through a cream separator. If a cream separator is unavailable, it is nearly impossible to obtain cream from the whole milk, because goat milk is naturally homogenized. Substitute cow cream.

3   pounds (1.36 g) pure vegetable shortening
17 ounces (482 g) extra-light olive oil
12 ounces (341 g) safflower oil
8   ounces (227 g) canola oil
1   pound (454 g, or approximately 2 cups) goat or cow cream, prepared as the milk was for soapmaking
2   pounds (908 g, or approximately 4 cups) goat or cow milk, prepared for soapmaking
12 ounces (340 g) pure sodium hydroxide (lye)
1   ounce (28.4 g) borax
¼   ounce (7.1 g) white sugar
¼   ounce (7.1 g) glycerin
½   ounce (14.2 g) peach fragrance

Special instruction. Add the cream to the milk before it is combined with the oils.

ROMANTIC ROSE
32 (4-ounce) bars

Delicate petals and the enchanting fragrance of roses enhance this romantic soap. It will appeal to those who are Victorian ladies at heart.

3 pounds (1.36 kg) pure vegetable shortening
17 ounces (482 g) extra light-olive oil
11 ounces (312 g) safflower oil
9 ounces (255 g) canola oil
3 pounds (1.36 kg, or approximately 6 cups) goat or cow milk, prepared for soapmaking
12 ounces (340 g) pure sodium hydroxide (lye)
1 ounce (28.4 g) borax
¼ ounce (7.1 g) white sugar
¼ ounce (7.1 g) glycerin
¾ cup (177 ml) dried or fresh red rose petals
½ ounce (14.2 g) rose fragrance oil

Special instruction. Add the rose petals and fragrance oil to the liquid mixture before it's run through the blender for the second time.

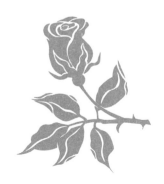

COCOA BUTTER SOAP
32 (4-ounce) bars

The tropical richness of cocoa butter blends delightfully with coconut and almond fragrances to create a bath bar that is rich and nourishing to your skin and soothing to the senses.

3	pounds (1.36 kg) pure vegetable shortening
17	ounces (482 g) extra-light olive oil
10	ounces (284 g) safflower oil
6	ounces (170 g) canola oil
4	ounces (113 g) cocoa butter
3	pounds (1.36 kg, or approximately 6 cups) goat or cow milk, prepared for soapmaking
12	ounces (340 g) pure sodium hydroxide (lye)
1	ounce (28.4 g) borax
¼	ounce (7.1 g) white sugar
¼	ounce (7.1 g) glycerin
½	ounce (14.2 g) almond fragrance
½	ounce (14.2 g) coconut fragrance oil

Special instructions. Melt the cocoa butter with the oils, and add the fragrance oil to the liquid mixture before it is run through the blender for the second time.

LAVENDER LACE

32 (4-ounce) bars

What fragrance could be more timeless than that of lavender? Lavender essence laces each bar, reminding one of gentler times and enduring innocence.

- 3 pounds (1.36 kg) pure vegetable shortening
- 17 ounces (482 g) extra-light olive oil
- 12 ounces (341 g) safflower oil
- 7 ounces (199 g) canola oil
- 3 pounds (1.36 kg, or approximately 6 cups) goat or cow milk, prepared for soapmaking
- 12 ounces (340 g) pure sodium hydroxide (lye)
- 1 ounce (28.4 g) borax
- ¼ ounce (7.1 g) white sugar
- ¼ ounce (7.1 g) glycerin
- ¾ cup (177 ml) dried lavender flowers
- 50 drops lavender essential oil

Special instructions. Add the dried lavender flowers to the liquid mixture when you run it through the blender for the first time. Add the lavender essential oil to the mixture when you run it through the blender for the second time.

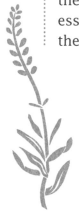

NITTY-GRITTY
32 (4-ounce) bars

Nothing cleans hard-working hands better than this super scrub soap made with ground eggshells. This is an excellent soap for mechanics, gardeners, painters, and anyone else who might need extra scrubbing power. The fragrance of cedar adds a nice touch.

3   pounds (1.36 kg) pure vegetable shortening
17   ounces (482 g) extra-light olive oil
12   ounces (341 g) safflower oil
7   ounces (199 g) canola oil
3   pounds (1.36 kg, or approximately 6 cups) goat or cow milk, prepared for soapmaking
12   ounces (340 g) pure sodium hydroxide (lye)
1   ounce (28.4 g) borax
¼   ounce (7.1 g) white sugar
¼   ounce (7.1 g) glycerin
¼   cup (59 ml) ground eggshells
50   drops cedar essential oil

Special instructions. In a blender, grind enough thoroughly dry eggshells (start with 1 dozen, but be ready to add more as needed) to make ¼ cup of finely ground eggshell powder. Add eggshells to the liquid mixture before it is run through the blender for the second time. Once the liquid soap mixture is poured into the mold, most of the ground eggshells will sink to the bottom, so after the bars are cut and cured, one side of them will be abrasive and the other side will be smooth.

HAPPY CAMPER
32 (4-ounce) bars

Folks who enjoy the outdoors will really appreciate Happy Camper soap, because it has a couple of natural bug repellents — citronella and eucalyptus oils — blended in. It really helps keep those bugs at bay!

 3 pounds (1.36 kg) pure vegetable shortening
17 ounces (482 g) extra-light olive oil
10 ounces (284 g) safflower oil
 7 ounces (199 g) canola oil
 3 pounds (1.36 kg, or approximately 6 cups) goat or cow milk, prepared for soapmaking
12 ounces (340 g) pure sodium hydroxide (lye)
 1 ounce (29.4 g) borax
 ¼ ounce (7.1 g) white sugar
 ¼ ounce (7.1 g) glycerin
 ½ ounce (14.2 g) citronella essential oil
 ¼ ounce (7.1 g) eucalyptus essential oil

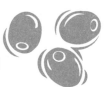

Special instruction. Add the essential oils to the liquid mixture the second time you run it through the blender.

ROSEMARY MIST

32 (4-ounce) bars

〰〰〰

This is an earthy soap with a lovely pale green color and the stimulating scent of rosemary.

3	pounds (1.36 kg) pure vegetable shortening
17	ounces (482 g) extra-light olive oil
10	ounces (284 g) safflower oil
7	ounces (199 g) canola oil
3	pounds (1.36 kg, or approximately 6 cups) goat or cow milk, prepared for soapmaking
12	ounces (340 g) pure sodium hydroxide (lye)
1	ounce (28.4 g) borax
¼	ounce (7.1 g) white sugar
¼	ounce (7.1 g) glycerin
⅓	cup (79 ml) dried rosemary
½	ounce (14.2 g) rosemary essential oil

Special instructions. Grate ⅓ cup of dried rosemary in the blender until it is a coarse powder. Add the rosemary to the liquid mixture the first time you run it through the blender. Add the rosemary essential oil to the liquid mixture the second time you run it through the blender.

CORNMEAL SCRUB

32 (4-ounce) bars

∿∿∿

Golden cornmeal makes this a soap with gentle abrasive qualities. Its golden color and fresh citrus smell make this a favorite soap to keep in the laundry room or around the kitchen sink for times when a quick scrub is needed!

3	pounds (1.36 kg) pure vegetable shortening
17	ounces (482 g) extra-light olive oil
10	ounces (284 g) safflower oil
8	ounces (227 g) canola oil
3	pounds (1.36 g, or approximately 6 cups) goat or cow milk, prepared for soapmaking
12	ounces (340 g) pure sodium hydroxide (lye)
1	ounce (28.4 g) borax
¼	ounce (7.1 g) white sugar
¼	ounce (7.1 g) glycerin
½	cup (118 ml) yellow cornmeal
¼	ounce (7.1 g) orange essential oil
¼	ounce (7.1 g) lemon essential oil

Special instructions. Add the cornmeal to the liquid mixture the first time you run it through the blender. Add the orange and lemon essential oils to the liquid the second time you run it through the blender.

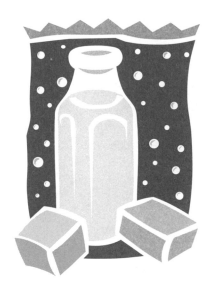

Recipes for
Other Milk-Based
Beauty Aids

CHAPTER 7

Pleasure is Nature's test, her sign of approval.
When man is happy, he is in harmony with himself and
his environment.

— Oscar Wilde

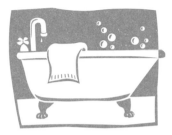

One of the finest ways to relax and pamper yourself is to indulge in one of Cleopatra's favorite pastimes, a rejuvenating, aromatic milk bath. A milk bath is a beneficial and relaxing beauty treatment for your whole body.

GENTLE, SOOTHING MILK BATHS

Milk baths have therapeutic value for several reasons. Milk gently softens and soothes dry, itchy skin. The natural lipids found in milk deeply moisturize the skin, and the moisture helps to accelerate skin cell renewal. The deep muscle relaxation and overall stress relief gained from a warm bath coupled with these moisturizing benefits make a milk bath a revitalizing treat!

How to take a milk bath is as important as the ingredients in the bath. Best is to shower first and wash your body with mild soap — using a homemade milk-based soap is a real complement to a milk bath! Be sure to rinse thoroughly. Massage moisturizing cream (either your favorite commercial brand or one of the excellent homemade versions in the next section) onto particularly dry skin areas. The warm bath will help your skin absorb the emollients from the applied cream before it rinses away. Wrap your clean hair in a towel and draw a very warm bath. Once the water reaches a desirable level, add one of the bath combinations below. Consider 20 minutes the minimum soaking time you'll need to derive the skin benefits of your bath; 40 minutes to an hour is even better.

Once you have finished your bath, you will gain maximum moisturizing benefits by simply rinsing yourself with a warm shower and toweling yourself gently dry. There is no need to "wash off" a milk bath using soap. Soap — even a gentle milk-based soap — would counteract the moisturizing benefits of your milk bath! Follow up immediately (before your skin is completely dry) with another application of moisturizer.

Here are some milk bath recipes to try. *Note:* Before you sink into that inviting bathwater, make sure your phone is unplugged and that the kids and the dog are safely occupied and have instructions not to knock on the door!

OBTAINING ESSENTIAL OILS

Look for essential oils at your local natural food store, gift shop, herb shop, or body-care shop. I've also included addresses for mail-order suppliers of essential oils in the resource list at the end of the book in case you find they are not available in your area.

GENTLE OATMEAL MILK BATH
1 bath

Especially good for dry, itchy skin.

¼ cup (59 ml) oatmeal
½ cup (118 ml) powdered cow or goat milk
1 tablespoon (15 ml) hazelnut oil
6 drops lavender essential oil

Put the oatmeal in a muslin bag (so it doesn't stick all over you or clog up your drain) and toss it into the bathwater. Add the milk and oils directly to the bathwater and mix well.

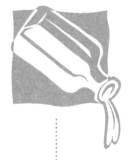

SOOTHING MILK SOAK
1 bath

Excellent for delicate skin.

2 cups (473 ml) powdered cow or goat milk
2 cups (473 ml) whole cow or goat milk
1 tablespoon (15 ml) almond oil
10 drops chamomile essential oil

Add all ingredients directly to bathwater and mix them well.

COCONUT-ALMOND MILK BATH
1 bath

Refreshing for all skin types.

3 cups (710 ml) powdered cow or goat milk
1 tablespoon (15 ml) almond oil
1 tablespoon (15 ml) coconut oil
3 drops pure vanilla extract
4 drops pure almond extract

Add all ingredients directly to bathwater and mix well. Pure enjoyment!

CREAMY MILK-BASED FACIALS

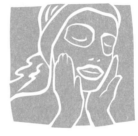

Facials are a gentle, effective way of cleansing, nourishing, and revitalizing the skin. Rich in emollients, milk-based facials are especially good because milk is a particularly effective moisturizer that leaves the skin feeling fresh and dewy. Once you have tried a milk-based facial for the first time, the healthy glow will speak for itself. Treat yourself to a creamy facial at least once a week . . . your skin will love you for it!

Moisturizers work most effectively when applied immediately after cleansing your skin, such as after a bath or a facial. Moisturizers help seal moisture into your skin, so be sure to slather plenty on dry skin areas of your body before you are completely dried off after your bath!

Because these cleansing creams and facials are freshly prepared and contain no harmful preservatives, they should be refrigerated and used within a week.

MORNING DEW CLEANSING CREAM
Approximately ¾ cup

Excellent for cleaning all skin types and smoothing small wrinkles.

3 tablespoons (45 ml) petroleum jelly
2 tablespoons (30 ml) beeswax
3 tablespoons (45 ml) mineral oil
1 tablespoon (15 ml) lemon juice
⅛ teaspoon (0.6 ml) borax
2 tablespoons (30 ml) whole cow milk
    or half-and-half
5 drops lemon essential oil
7 drops chamomile essential oil

Over low heat, melt the petroleum jelly and beeswax together. Gradually add the mineral oil and blend until there is no separation. In a separate container, warm the lemon juice over low heat. Stir in the borax until it is dissolved, then carefully add to the wax mixture and blend thoroughly until creamy. Whisk in the milk and essential oils and blend until cool. Spoon into a clean jar, label and date it, and store in the refrigerator.

To use, apply generously with fingertips, wait 4 to 8 minutes, and gently wipe off the excess with a cotton ball.

CREAMY RICH MOISTURIZING CREAM
Approximately ¾ cup

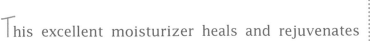

This excellent moisturizer heals and rejuvenates the skin.

3   tablespoons (45 ml) petroleum jelly
2   tablespoons (30 ml) beeswax
1   tablespoon (15 ml) lanolin
2   teaspoons (10 ml) almond oil
1   teaspoon (5 ml) wheat germ oil
½   teaspoon (2.5 ml) glycerin
2   tablespoons (30 ml) warm (not hot) whole cow milk
    or half-and-half
1   tablespoon (15 ml) strong comfrey infusion
    (see box on page 84)
¼   teaspoon (1.3 ml) borax
6   drops almond essential oil or jasmine essential oil

Melt the petroleum jelly, beeswax, and lanolin over low heat until blended. Remove from heat and add the almond and wheat germ oils and glycerin, blending together until creamy. Dissolve the borax in the warm milk, add the comfrey infusion, and slowly whisk the milk mixture into the cream. Keep stirring and as the entire mixture is cooling, slowly add the essential oil. Once the mixture is cool and thick, store in a labeled jar in the refrigerator for up to 1 week. This is a perfect moisturizer to use after a milk bath!

BLOSSOMS AND BUTTERMILK CLEANSING MILK

Approximately ¾ cup

Soothing and nourishing for all skin types, and especially for dry or delicate skin.

- ½ cup (118 ml) buttermilk
- 2 tablespoons (30 ml) dried calendula (healing for dry or damaged skin)
- 2 tablespoons (30 ml) dried parsley (excellent conditioner for sensitive skin)

Warm the buttermilk over low heat until it is warm to touch. Remove from heat and add the calendula and parsley. Cover and let sit for 1 hour, then strain and refrigerate. Use within 1 week. To apply, dab on with a cotton ball and rinse off with lukewarm water.

MAKING AN HERBAL INFUSION

An infusion is a strong water-based preparation that is similar in nature to tea. To prepare an infusion, fill a quart jar halfway (more or less, depending on the strength of the infusion desired) with dried or fresh plant material and cover with water that has been brought to a boil. Cover and let stand for several hours, strain, and store in a labeled glass jar in the refrigerator for up to 2 weeks.

Recommended Herbs for Infusions:

Comfrey. Excellent for all skin types. Comfrey is renowned for its ability to speed up cell regeneration.

Nettle leaf. Rich in nutrients, nettle leaf nourishes the skin.

Burdock. Infusing burdock produces an invigorating skin tonic that soothes problem dry skin types.

Raspberry leaf. Contains many important vitamins such as A, B complex, and C along with minerals and potassium. Tones and refreshes the skin.

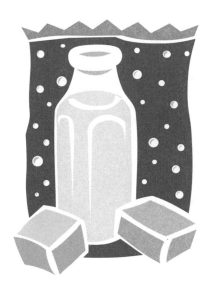

Package It
with Appeal

CHAPTER

8

Man is always more than he can know of himself, consequently his accomplishments, time and again, will come as a surprise to him.

— Golo Mann

Once you get started as a soapmaker, you'll soon find yourself making more soap than you or your family can use. Luckily, soap makes a wonderful and unusual handmade gift. Beautiful and gentle milk-based soap is a gift the lucky recipient will remember long after the bar is used up!

And if you've made the leap into selling your soap, keep in mind that handmade soap is more often purchased as a gift item than for personal use.

Whether you plan to sell your soap or give it away as gifts, the manner in which you present it will determine its success as much or more than the quality of the soap itself. Packaging your gift or product in an appealing, eye-catching manner is important. Good packaging reflects the quality of your product. You will want your packaging to convey the charm and uniqueness that cannot be found in commercially purchased soap.

If you're selling your soap, good packaging also justifies the price you will be charging. You cannot expect consumers to pay $4.00 for a bar of soap carelessly wrapped in a piece of plastic. But imagine that same bar of soap wrapped in pretty calico fabric and tied with a satin ribbon, and suddenly you have a $4.00 item. A good presentation of your soap speaks well of you as the producer.

Remember, soap must be cured for a minimum of 6 weeks before wrapping. On the other hand, it has no expiration date!

Wrapping Ideas

Be creative in your packaging. Your gift soaps will be enjoyed and treasured all the more by their recipients. And if you sell your soaps, a good impression will increase your marketing success and win you a good reputation.

Creative packaging ideas to try include:

◆ Wrap the soap in calico fabric and tie it with a satin ribbon. If you're selling your soap, wrap each variety in the same way for easy identification.

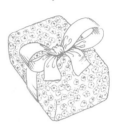

◆ Roll up a solid-colored washcloth or hand towel and tie a fabric-wrapped bar of soap to it with raffia.

◆ Fold a pretty kitchen washcloth and tie an unwrapped bar of soap to it with a long piece of raffia. With a hot-glue gun, glue a star anise in the center of the bow.

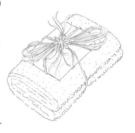

◆ Purchase pretty country-type mugs at close-out sales, put about 1 inch (2.5 cm) of fine curled wood shavings (sometimes sold as "excelsior") in the bottom, place a bar of soap in the mug, and tie a raffia bow to the handle.

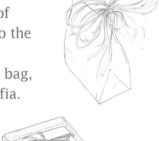

◆ Put bar of soap in small brown paper bag, fold top, punch hole, and tie with raffia.

◆ Make small wooden crates that hold two bars of soap snugly and tie them in with raffia.

◆ Make wooden soap dishes and tie a bar of soap onto each one with raffia.

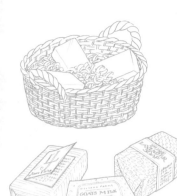

- ◆ Purchase inexpensive baskets, put 1 inch (2.5 cm) of fine colored wood shavings in the bottom, and place two or three soaps in them.
- ◆ Purchase (or make your own!) hand-made paper, wrap bars, and add your own handmade label.

WHAT'S IN A NAME?

As you gain experience and proficiency in soapmaking, you will want to experiment with different soap recipes. Whether as gifts or for sale, your soaps will have a special feel if each variety has a distinctive name. Let your creativity loose when naming your handcrafted soaps!

For example, maybe you noticed in the recipe chapter that I gave each soap a name. Instead of blandly naming the soap for campers Camping Soap, I called it Happy Camper. The first name has a very utilitarian ring to it — not catchy or cute, just functional. But take that bar of soap, wrap it in camouflage fabric with the tag HAPPY CAMPER, and it will leave a striking impression and practically sell itself.

The same is true of Lavender Lace and Romantic Rose. Their names are delightful and alluring compared to dull names like Rose Soap or Lavender Soap. Some soaps, like Oatmeal and Cocoa Butter, can easily stand up under a plain name, but it never hurts to use your imagination to create a catchier one.

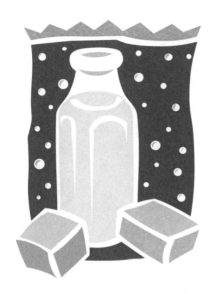

Making Soap,
Making Money

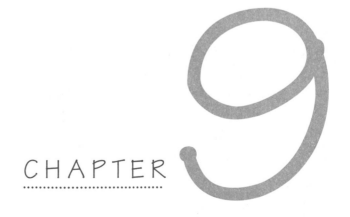

CHAPTER

Money is like a sixth sense without which you cannot make complete use of the other five.
— W. Somerset Maugham, *Of Human Bondage*

As you gain experience and proficiency in soap-making, your entrepreneurial instincts may awaken. If they do, you will find that you have chosen a hobby that has the potential to make money. Handmade soap has real possibilities as a product that can be marketed with a high profit margin and excellent consumer appeal. There is new and insatiable consumer interest in handmade soaps of all kinds. Milk soaps are particularly popular because they are unusual and especially kind to delicate complexions.

Creating a market for your soap starts with evaluating the quality of your product. You'll find an excellent test group for your soap's appeal right in your own family. As a new soapmaker, you will need to use your product personally so that you have honest and convincing selling points to convey to potential customers. Spend your first year making as much soap as time allows. Use it yourself, and decide what you like about your soap and where improvements could be made. Give it as gifts to friends and family, and encourage them, too, to evaluate it. Try out different ideas for recipes and packaging your soap.

Before you try to sell your soap, be sure it's of high quality. A small percentage of handmade soap for sale lacks quality and workmanship. A fast dollar is never as important as a stable reputation. Consumers will spend top dollar on products of superior craftsmanship. Repeat business is the real bread and butter when selling your soap. A satisfied customer always comes back, and usually brings a friend!

SETTING A PRICE

Don't make the mistake of trying to price your soap to be competitive with commercially manufactured soaps. Handmade soaps are in a class of their own. They boast unique characteristics that are nonexistent in commercial soaps and can thus command a higher price. Once you establish what will characterize your soaps, you will be able to extol those credits as strong selling points. Honesty should be your first premise, always. Don't expound upon what doesn't exist — but do, as much as it pertains to your soap, confidently convey enthusiasm for your product. If you are excited about your soap, other people will be, too.

Figure Production Costs

How much should you charge for a bar of soap? Let's first figure out what it costs to make a batch of soap. While prices will vary greatly, we'll use the following rough figures:

COST OF PRODUCING 1 BATCH OF SOAP

1½ quarts goat milk @ $3.00 per quart	$4.50
One 12-ounce can of lye	$1.50
3 pounds vegetable shortening	$4.00
17 ounces extra-light olive oil	$3.00
12 ounces safflower oil	$1.75
7 ounces canola oil	$1.00
½ ounce glycerin	$1.00
½ ounce white sugar	$ .20
1 ounce borax	$ .15
Silicone bakery paper (3 sheets @ $ .50 a sheet)	$1.50
Fragrance	$1.00
Total Cost	**$19.60**

For this batch of soap, your costs are $19.60. This does not include costs of molds and equipment, because those are considered starting business expenses and those are one-time purchases. We are also not including an hourly rate for your work in producing the soap, nor the costs of marketing your products (discussed in the next section). For now, simply look at what the basic potential profit margin in a batch of soap is by comparing ingredient costs with potential selling price. To get the complete picture of your business's break-even point, you'll have to include equipment, time, and marketing costs in your calculations, spreading the equipment costs out over perhaps a year's worth of soap production.

Now divide the cost of ingredients for a typical batch of soap, $19.60, by the number of bars you typically get from a batch, 32: $19.60 ÷ 32 = $.61, giving approximately 61 cents as your cost per bar of soap. You will probably wrap each individual bar, so let's add a rough cost of about 25 cents per bar (this is somewhat high and could cover the expense of wrapping your soap in fabric and adding a satin tie): $.25 + $.61 = $.86. Thus, each bar of soap will cost you about 86 cents to produce.

Research the Competition

After figuring your costs, a good frame of reference for gauging prices is to find out what other soapmakers charge for their products. Most home-based soap companies will send out a catalog on request. (Many require a modest fee. It is a gesture of respect to honor that request. If you don't, most will send you a catalog anyway, but if you don't make a purchase, the costs of the catalog and postage become a loss to the business.) As you review these catalogs, pay attention to the weight of each bar of soap as well as its price. You will find quite a broad price range, depending on both the company and the type of soap it is selling. This should help you find your price niche.

I have found that a safe midrange price for hand-crafted soap is $1.00 per ounce. This works nicely if you are producing the 32 (4-ounce) bars of soap as described in the recipes I offer. You could charge as much as $4.00 per bar (even though the bars cure down to 3½ ounces), and receive $4.00 x 32 = $128.00 per batch. Offering a price break on volume purchases can also be an incentive to the consumer. Something like three bars for $10.50 would offer the customer a savings of 50 cents per bar. Instead of seeing that as a loss of profit, you can look at it as soap you may not have otherwise sold. Everyone loves a bargain!

Now let's subtract the cost per bar, $.86, from the $4.00 per bar selling price: ($4.00 - $.86 = $3.14). Thus, you will see a profit of $3.14 per bar. Even if you offer volume incentives that reduce your selling price to $3.50 per bar, you still show a profit of $2.64. Any businessperson will tell you that a profit margin of over 250 percent is quite respectable. Of course, there will be other costs to consider, as well as ways to trim these listed, but this gives you a general idea of what to expect and maybe even a little incentive to boot!

MARKETING YOUR SOAP

Where do find places to sell your soap? After you do a little searching you will be surprised at how many places you will find, including crafts shows and shops, museum stores, and mail-order sales.

Crafts Shows

Reserving a space at local crafts shows is an excellent way to start marketing your soap, especially just after Thanksgiving, when shoppers are looking for unique gifts for the upcoming holiday season. Contact area chambers of commerce for a list of upcoming crafts shows. Crafts shows usually sell out their spaces early and quickly, so plan ahead. Make sure the shows you get involved with feature handmade craft items only. Bazaars and flea markets are not the kinds of places where you will sell much soap, because they attract a different kind of consumer from those that crafts shows do.

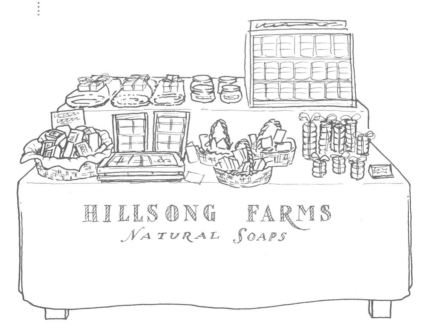

Spend some time planning a creative, eye-catching display.

Set up your display at home to get a feel for how you can arrange your soaps and gift sets to make everything look appealing and eye-catching. Some crafts shows provide tables and chairs, others do not. If the show you are interested in is being held outside, you will need a canopy tent, tables, and chairs. Other useful items to have on hand include:

- **Calculator** to calculate purchase totals and tax.
- **Change box** with at least $50.00 in small change, including lots of $1.00 bills and quarters.
- **Receipt book.** Customers prefer to see their purchases itemized, and this gives you an accurate record of your sales.
- **Pens.** Bring along several, since they tend to walk off!
- **Business cards.** These are a handy and economical way to advertise your soapmaking business. Your business cards should be eye-catching, and you should carry them around and tack them up on every information board you find to help the public become familiar with your product.
- **Customized stamp with your business name, and stamp pad.** Stamping receipts and bags with your name and phone number is a great way to get customers to remember you and come back for more.
- **Bags.** Soaps are small, so you can use small paper lunch bags; colored lunch bags are especially cute. Whatever size paper bag you use, be sure to stamp your business name and address on it, since this is free advertising. A nice touch is to wrap the purchase loosely in colored tissue paper with a little of the tissue paper pulled out of the top of the bag. Fold over one corner of the

bag, punch through the fold using a hole puncher, run a little piece of raffia through the hole, and tie it into a bow. Customers really enjoy these kinds of pretty extra touches, and they help leave a lasting good impression of your business.

- **Display racks.** Go to several crafts shows and look at what exhibitors are using to display their products. You will find that the vast assortment of creative ways crafters display their wares will inspire ideas of your own. You can purchase ready-made display racks that will fit on your table, or create them yourself.
- **Supply box.** This should include items such as tape, string, scissors, glue, paper, ribbon, tacks, and anything else you think would be handy to have packed for an unforeseen emergency.
- **Guest book.** Have your customers sign your guest book so you can start to compile a mailing list; this will help you establish a mail-order business.

This list should help you get started in exhibiting at crafts shows. Certainly you will add to this list as you gain experience as an exhibitor.

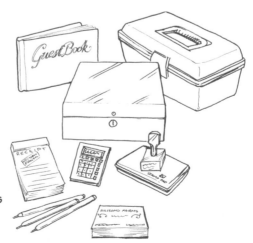

Organize all the supplies you will need.

Mail-Order Sales

Selling by mail order is very convenient for both you and the customer. It allows you to make money selling your product without having to leave your home. Likewise, your customer does not have to wait to meet you at another crafts show to make purchases.

When working with mail orders, remember to add a shipping and handling charge. If the order is large, you have the option of waiting until your customer's check clears at your bank before sending out the merchandise.

Since handmade soaps make such great gifts, you can offer to mail purchases directly to a gift recipient. You may want to offer extras such as gift wrapping and the enclosure of a small card with a message from the sender.

If the prospect of mail-order sales sounds interesting, the first step is to develop a small brochure to advertise your soaps, including a simple order form. This is where you should really shine with enthusiasm for your product. In a few short paragraphs, you have to convey to potential buyers what makes your product is unique, what makes it great, and why it is an excellent purchase choice. If writing comes easily to you, this will be a fun project. If you feel you could use help, enlist a good friend or family member who has a knack for creative writing. Then submit your rough draft to a reputable print shop, and it will produce your brochures.

Advertising in magazines and newsletters that feature back-to-basics, country-life topics is also an avenue to investigate. Check each magazine for key information such as circulation numbers: How many prospective readers will your ad reach? Consider also that a one-time ad will not generate the kind of interest you are looking for. Consumers are more affected by ads that become familiar by appearing regularly. You will have to decide if you will make back the money you spend on buying ad space, let alone sell enough to generate a profit. If you take this route, make sure ordering information is clearly stated in your ad. Adding a simple order form can help move potential customers to act.

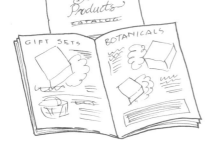

A small, personally written brochure promotes mail-order business.

THE LEGALITIES OF SELLING SOAP

Before you jump into the soap industry, be sure to check the federal regulations and any state regulations that might affect you. One important federal regulation is the distinction between a soap and a cosmetic. There are much stricter federal Food and Drug Administration (FDA) regulations for packaging, labeling, and sales of cosmetics, so be careful not to make any healing or medicinal claims for your soap, or it will fall into the cosmetic realm. So, despite what you might think, don't advertise the fact that your soap "makes older skin look younger." Let the users discover this beauty secret for themselves.

Crafts Shops

Consider consigning your soaps to crafts shops. This is a great way to sell your product without a lot of effort. Crafts shops charge a commission, usually between 30 and 40 percent. This covers many costs that you as a consignor do not have to concern yourself with. A storefront shop has the overhead costs of insurance, advertising, electricity, payroll, supplies, and much more to cover. Keep this in mind if the commission seems high to you. The shop is doing the work of attracting customers for you; all you have to do is supply the product. With soap, your profit margin is high enough that you should not consider increasing your selling prices to cover the shop's commission. Your product will not do you any good sitting on a shelf overpriced and unpurchased.

Museum Shops

Museums are another place that might be interested in featuring your soaps to sell, because of the historical interest in early handcrafts. They will probably charge a commission comparable to what gift shops charge.

Museums may also give you the opportunity to offer workshops about soapmaking, and this will expand local awareness of your soapmaking business. If you do get an opportunity to teach a workshop or display your soap for an event associated with a museum, consider dressing in period costume. The public is always thrilled by this sort of visual image, and it helps people to better relate to the history you may be speaking about. Costuming will lend an air of credibility and character that will be long remembered. And make sure you set out business cards and brochures for people to take!

Successfully marketing your soap can provide a modest source of part-time income. It is very rewarding to have people purchase and enjoy soap that you have handcrafted. In time, not only will you be making money but you also will be making new friends by meeting people who admire what you do and enjoy the product you produce.

RESOURCE INFORMATION

Knowledge is of two kinds. We know a subject ourselves, or we know where we can find information.

— Samuel Johnson

Goat Milk

Fresh and powdered goat milk is available in many supermarkets and natural food stores across the country. To locate dairy-goat breeders in your area, contact the following organization:

American Dairy Goat Association
209 West Main Street
P.O. Box 865
Spindale, NC 28160
(704) 286-3801
www.adga.org

Other Supplies

Aroma Vera
5310 Beethoven Street
Los Angeles, CA 90066
(800) 669-9514
www.aromavera.com
Pure, high-quality essential oils and aromatherapy-related products.

Aromaland
1326 Rufina Circle
Santa Fe, NM 87501-2927
(800) 933-5267
www.aromaland.com
Pure, high-quality essential oils and aromatherapy-related products.

The Essential Oil Company
8225 SE 7th Avenue
Portland, OR 97202
(800) 729-5912
(503) 872-8772 in Oregon
www.essentialoil.com
Pure, high-quality essential oils and aromatherapy-related products.

From Nature With Love
P.O. Box 201
Hawleyville, CT 06440
www.fromnaturewithlove.com

Frontier Co-op Herbs
3021 78th Street
P.O. Box 299
Norway, IA 52318
(800) 669-3275
www.frontiercoop.com
Wide variety of essential oils, bulk herbs, and vegetable oils. Company direct business/wholesale accounts only. Joining your local community co-op may allow you to make wholesale purchases, as most co-ops have business accounts with Frontier.

The Herb Companion
Ogden Publications
1503 SW 42nd Street
Topeka, KS 66609
(800) 456-5835
www.discoverherbs.com
Magazine advertising variety of herbal suppliers.

Lavender Lane
7337 #1 Roseville Road
Sacramento, CA 95842
(888) 593-4400
www.lavenderlane.com
Carries hard-to-find herbalware; bottles, droppers, essential oils, and labels.

Liberty Natural Products, Inc.
8120 SE Stark
Portland, OR 97215
(800) 289-8427
www.libertynatural.com

Mountain Rose Herbs
85472 Dilley Lane
Eugene, OR 97405
(800) 879-3337
www.mountainroseherbs.com
Dried herbs.

Original Swiss Aromatics
Pacific Institute of Aromatherapy
P.O. Box 6723
San Rafael, CA 94903
(415) 459-3998
www.originalswissaromatics.com

Pretty Baby Herbal Soap Co.
P.O. Box 555
China Grove, NC 28023
(800) 673-8167
Soapmaking kits.

The Soap Saloon
4500-C Beloit Drive
Sacramento, CA 95838
(916) 334-4894
www.soapsaloon.com

The Soap Shoppe
P.O. Box 162
Mikado, MI 48745
(517) 736-6583
Essential oils, tinctures, potpourri fragrances, extruded vinyl soap molds, soapmaking supplies and kits, silicone bakery paper, more.

Star-West Botanicals
11253 Trade Center Drive
Rancho Cordova, CA 95742
(888) 369-4372
www.starwestbotanicals.com
Offers an excellent selection of dried herbs, essential oils, fragrances, and more. Business/ wholesale accounts only. You may be able to order their products through your local co-op.

Storey Publishing
210 MASS MoCA Way
North Adams, MA 01247
(800) 441-5700
www.storey.com
Soapmaking books.

Summers Past Farms
15602 Old Highway 80
Flinn Springs, CA 92021
(619) 390-1523
www.summerspastfarms.com
Soapmaking kit.

Sunfeather Herbal Soap Co.
1551 State Highway 72
Potsdam, NY 13676
(315) 265-3648
www.sunsoap.com
Complete line of soapmaking supplies.

INDEX

OTHER STOREY TITLES YOU WILL ENJOY

The Essential Oils Book, by Colleen K. Dodt. Discusses the many uses of aromatherapy and its applications in everyday life. 160 pages. Paperback. ISBN 0-88266-913-3.

Making Natural Liquid Soaps, by Catherine Failor. Create all-natural, inexpensive hand soaps, shampoos, shower gels, bubble baths, and more. 144 pages. Paperback. ISBN 1-58017-243-1.

Making Transparent Soap, by Catherine Failor. Produce transparent soaps that are milder, richer, and creamier than any commercial soap on the market. 144 pages. Paperback. ISBN 1-58017-244-X.

Melt & Mold Soap Crafting, by C. Kaila Westeman. Cook soaps in the microwave! Use a meltable glycerin soap base and readily available colorants and fragrances to design works of soap art. 144 pages. Paperback. ISBN 1-58017-293-8.

Natural BabyCare, by Colleen K. Dodt. Offers recipes for creating natural personal care items for babies and features on self-care during pregnancy and child birth. 160 pages. Paperback. ISBN 0-88266-953-2.

The Natural Soap Book, by Susan Miller Cavitch. Provides basic vegetable-based soap recipes along with ideas on scenting, coloring, trimming, and wrapping soaps. 192 pages. Paperback. ISBN 0-88266-888-9.

The Soapmaker's Companion, by Susan Miller Cavitch. Presents the most authoritative handbook for making natural, vegetable-based soaps in a range of styles. 288 Pages. Paperback. ISBN 0-88266-965-6.

These and other books from Storey Publishing are available wherever books are sold or by calling 1-800-441-5700.
Visit us at www.storey.com.